Nourish Without Nonsense

#GoingBackToTheRoots

Saanchi Shetty

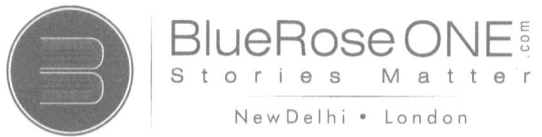

BLUEROSE PUBLISHERS
India | U.K.

Copyright © Saanchi Shetty 2025

All rights reserved by author. No part of this publication may be reproduced, stored in a retrieval system or transmitted in any form or by any means, electronic, mechanical, photocopying, recording or otherwise, without the prior permission of the author. Although every precaution has been taken to verify the accuracy of the information contained herein, the publisher assumes no responsibility for any errors or omissions. No liability is assumed for damages that may result from the use of information contained within.

BlueRose Publishers takes no responsibility for any damages, losses, or liabilities that may arise from the use or misuse of the information, products, or services provided in this publication.

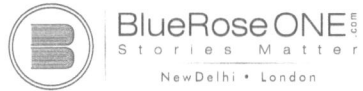

For permissions requests or inquiries regarding this publication,
please contact:

BLUEROSE PUBLISHERS
www.BlueRoseONE.com
info@bluerosepublishers.com
+91 8882 898 898
+4407342408967

ISBN: 978-93-7018-762-7

Cover design: Lovina Madhav
Typesetting: Namrata Saini

First Edition: May 2025

Preface

I was around five years old when my struggles with digestive issues began—constipation, bloating, and persistent stomach discomfort were constant parts of my life. This was surprising, considering I came from a family where health and nutrition were held in the highest regard. "Ghar ka khana" was seen as the ultimate solution to all ailments, and yet, my body didn't seem to align with this conventional wisdom. My parents, like many in Indian households, believed that home-cooked meals made from fresh ingredients were all one needed for good health. But for me, something always felt off.

My mornings started before sunrise, often at 4:35 AM, filled with intense training sessions in basketball and track running. I was always an active child, excelling in sports and fitness. Despite my rigorous physical routine, my gut health remained a persistent problem, refusing to improve even with disciplined eating. Like most Indian households, my diet consisted of the so-called pillars of good health—rotis, vegetables, milk, and protein. The elders in my family would always say, "Eat more, and you'll grow stronger." But my body wasn't cooperating. Instead of feeling energized and nourished, I felt sluggish and unwell.

Over the years, I visited numerous doctors and hospitals, desperately searching for relief. From well-known specialists to alternative medicine practitioners, I explored every possible solution. I was prescribed every remedy imaginable—fiber supplements, probiotics, digestive enzymes, ayurvedic medicines, homeopathic treatments, and even expensive allopathic medications. Yet, nothing seemed to make a lasting difference. Doctors reassured me that my diet was fine and that these were "normal digestive issues" that I would eventually outgrow. But deep down, I knew that this wasn't normal. I had learned to live with these issues, until everything worsened after I gave birth to my daughter.

Motherhood is a transformative experience, both physically and emotionally. While I was prepared for sleepless nights and a new routine, I wasn't prepared for the drastic impact childbirth would have on my body. My digestion, which had always been a problem, became even worse. I was constantly bloated, fatigued, and dealing with unpredictable stomach issues. Despite my best efforts to regain control of my health, nothing seemed to work. The same advice echoed everywhere I went: "Eat more rotis, more vegetables, more milk, more protein." But the more I followed this traditional advice, the worse I felt.

Determined to find a solution, I tried it all—low-calorie diets, trendy fad diets, anything that promised quick results. I did manage to lose weight post-pregnancy, but only through hours at the gym, not because of any dietary recommendation that was supposed to help. My relationship with food became increasingly strained. I viewed food as a problem rather than a source of nourishment. Frustration and exhaustion took over. The constant cycle of medications and restrictive diets wasn't working. I knew there had to be another way.

That's when I took matters into my own hands and started researching gut health. I read books, attended seminars, and followed the latest scientific studies. I learned about the impact of food intolerances, gut microbiome imbalances, and how diet plays a crucial role in overall well-being. This led to a breakthrough—what if gluten and dairy were the culprits all along? What if my body had been reacting negatively to them for years, but I had ignored the signs because they were considered "healthy" foods?

Skeptical yet hopeful, I decided to eliminate gluten and dairy from my diet. Within weeks, I noticed a dramatic shift. My bloating reduced significantly, my energy levels improved, and for the first time in years, I felt lighter and healthier. The transformation was undeniable. My skin cleared up, my metabolism improved, and my digestive system functioned better than ever before.

That was the turning point. What began as an attempt to heal my gut evolved into something bigger — a newfound understanding of nutrition and how food affects overall well-being. It was no longer just about avoiding discomfort; it became about reclaiming my health in a way that felt natural and sustainable. I realized that health isn't about deprivation or extreme dieting. It's about making choices that work for your body, rather than following outdated nutritional beliefs.

As I delved deeper into the world of nutrition, I was shocked by how much misinformation exists around food and health. Modern nutrition has been tangled in trends, marketing gimmicks, and extreme diet rules, making the simple act of eating well feel complicated and overwhelming. From detox teas and fat-burning supplements to calorie-counting apps and restrictive meal plans, the health industry has turned wellness into a business, preying on people's insecurities and confusion.

But in reality, nutrition is straightforward. It's about listening to your body, nourishing it with the right foods, and making choices that support long-term health without stress or confusion. The more I learned, the more I realized that much of what we are told about food is influenced by marketing rather than actual science. For example, we are led to believe that dairy is essential for strong bones, yet many people (myself included) experience adverse effects from it. We are told that whole wheat is the healthiest option, yet for those with gluten sensitivities, it can be highly inflammatory. The more I questioned these so-called "truths," the more clarity I gained about what real health looks like.

I've always believed in the power of ancestral wisdom when it comes to food. The way our ancestors thrived on whole foods, the simplicity of their meals, and their intuitive connection with nature deeply resonate with me. But somewhere along the way, we've lost that wisdom — replacing wholesome, natural food with processed alternatives, additives, and rigid diet culture. Instead of honoring our body's needs, we force ourselves into one-size-fits-all dietary trends that do more harm than good.

This book is my way of helping people rediscover the joy in eating and living well. I want people to feel catered to and nurtured, to embrace a healthy lifestyle rather than resent it. It's not about following unrealistic meal plans or spending hours counting calories — it's about making mindful choices, finding balance, and most importantly, enjoying the process of nourishing yourself. True wellness isn't about restriction; it's about understanding what works best for your body and making peace with food.

Nourish Without Nonsense is not about making health an exhausting, all-consuming pursuit. Instead, it's about understanding your body, trusting your instincts, and making small, consistent changes that lead to lifelong wellness. I want to simplify nutrition for those who feel overwhelmed by conflicting advice. I want to provide practical, sustainable solutions that make healthy eating accessible, enjoyable, and freeing.

My hope is that through this book, you will gain the clarity and confidence to take control of your health — without the nonsense, without the confusion, and without the stress. Whether you're struggling with digestive issues, feeling lost in a sea of diet trends, or simply looking to improve your overall well-being, this book is here to guide you. It's not about perfection; it's about progress.

Welcome to Nourish Without Nonsense — where wellness meets simplicity, and health is a journey, not a punishment.

Contents

Introducing 1

Healthy Lifestyle 5

Morning Routine: Setting the Tone for a Healthier Day 13

High-Fiber, High-Protein Breakfast: Fuel for Champions (and Regular Humans) 26

The Midday Meal—Finding Balance in Lunch 43

The Snack Debate - When, What, and How Much? 66

Dinner - The Final Meal of the Day 79

Carbs: The Good, The Bad, and the Delicious 100

Protein: The Mighty Macronutrient 108

Fats – The Forgotten Heroes of Nutrition 117

Water – The Elixir of Life (and Also Your Best Friend) 127

Fibre – Your Gut's Best Friend (and Yours Too) 138

Beverages: The Liquid Side of Life 148

Diet Dilemmas: The Battle of the Diets (And Which One Might Actually Work for You) 165

Understanding the Circadian Rhythm – The Body's Natural Clock 187

Detox and Fasting – The Ancient Art of Saying No to Food 207

Gut: The Unsung Hero of Your Health 230

Introducing

Nourish Without Nonsense

For years, we've been bombarded with conflicting advice about food, health, and what it truly means to nourish our bodies. One day, carbohydrates are the enemy; the next, fats take the blame. Detox teas, miracle diets, and fasting fads flood our screens, each promising quick fixes and effortless transformations. Yet, despite all the information available, many people still feel lost, confused, and disconnected from their own health. Why? Because we've overcomplicated something that should be simple.

As a nutrition and lifestyle guide for the past two decades, I, Saanchi Shetty, have seen every diet trend come and go. I've worked with clients who've tried everything—keto, paleo, juice cleanses, intermittent fasting—only to find themselves frustrated, exhausted, and often worse off than before. The truth is, nutrition isn't about deprivation or extremes. It's about balance, sustainability, and understanding what your body truly needs.

Why This Book?

Nourish Without Nonsense was born out of a need to cut through the clutter and bring clarity to the world of nutrition. This book is not about following rigid rules or punishing yourself for enjoying food. Instead, it's about equipping you with the knowledge to make informed, realistic, and enjoyable choices that align with your health goals.

In this book, we'll break down complex nutritional concepts into simple, actionable steps. We'll explore how food affects your gut health, metabolism, hormones, and energy levels—without diving into pseudoscience or overwhelming medical jargon. Whether you're looking to improve digestion, detoxify naturally, or simply feel more energized, this book will guide you toward a lifestyle that works for *you* — not against you.

The Problem with Modern Nutrition Trends

One of the biggest issues with today's approach to nutrition is the obsession with quick fixes. We've all seen those "lose 10 pounds in a week" diets or "miracle detox drinks" that claim to flush out toxins overnight. But here's the reality — our bodies are already designed to detoxify naturally. Your liver, kidneys, gut, and skin are working every day to eliminate waste and maintain balance. The problem arises when we overload these systems with poor nutrition, excessive stress, and unhealthy habits.

Extreme detoxes and aggressive fasting methods can do more harm than good, often leading to nutrient deficiencies, slowed metabolism, and hormonal imbalances. Instead of jumping from one diet trend to another, we need to focus on sustainable habits that support our body's natural functions.

The Role of this Book in Your Nutrition

At its core, this book encourages you to return to your roots — to eat the way your ancestors did, to sync your meals with your circadian rhythm, and to nourish your gut for overall health. It sheds light on why modern diets often fail, why gut health is at the center of everything, and how small, mindful changes in your eating habits can create a profound impact on your energy levels, metabolism, and overall well-being.

A Balanced Approach to Fasting and Detox

Fasting has gained popularity for its potential benefits, from weight management to cellular repair. However, many people dive into fasting too aggressively, leading to fatigue, irritability, and even metabolic damage. Here, you'll learn how to ease into fasting safely, choosing methods that fit your lifestyle and health needs. Whether it's intermittent fasting, time-restricted eating, or mindful detox practices, this book will help you approach fasting in a way that enhances rather than harms your well-being.

Mindful Eating: The Key to Long-Term Success

Diet culture has trained us to fear food, count calories obsessively, and view eating as a battle. But what if we shifted our mindset? What if we started seeing food as nourishment rather than numbers? Mindful eating is about listening to your body's hunger and fullness cues, enjoying meals without guilt, and making choices that truly serve your health.

This book won't tell you to eliminate entire food groups or label foods as "good" or "bad." Instead, we'll focus on balance — choosing whole, nutrient-dense foods while still allowing room for the foods you love. Because true nourishment isn't just about what you eat — it's about how you eat and the relationship you build with food.

What You'll Learn in This Book

Throughout *Nourish Without Nonsense*, we'll dive into:

✓ *How to start your morning and dive into your day?*

✓ *What kinds of nutrients are needed for your body to be healthy and happy?*

✓ *The science of detox and why your body doesn't need extreme cleanses*

✓ *How to support your gut for better digestion, immunity, and overall health*

✓ *Sustainable fasting methods that enhance, rather than deplete, your body*

✓ *The role of hydration, movement, and sleep in natural detoxification*

✓ *Practical strategies to develop a balanced, guilt-free relationship with food*

Metabolism, inflammation, insulin resistance and hormones

A Final Word Before We Begin

Health is not a one-size-fits-all journey. What works for one person may not work for another, and that's okay. This book isn't about prescribing rigid rules—it's about empowering you with the knowledge to make the best choices for *your* body.

As you read through these pages, keep an open mind and be willing to experiment. Small, consistent changes lead to lasting results. You don't need to overhaul your entire diet overnight; you just need to take the first step.

So, if you're ready to ditch the nonsense, embrace nourishment, and finally feel *good* about your food choices—let's get started.

Healthy Lifestyle

Food is powerful. It's the superhero your body needs — minus the cape, but trust me, it's just as effective. Every bite you take is like a secret weapon for your organs, helping them fight off the villains of poor health. Think of it this way: your heart's the captain of the team, your brain's the strategist, and your stomach's the overworked intern. They all need the right fuel to keep you winning. So, let's get started on how to turn cluelessness into confidence and make those 80% of problems go "puff" like magic.

Your body is basically an incredibly complicated machine that didn't come with a manual. Each organ has its job, and together they form an Avengers-style team that's fighting for your survival. Give them junk food, and it's like handing Thor a rubber mallet. Feed them wholesome, nutrient-rich foods, and suddenly everyone's pulling their weight. You don't need to memorize nutrition textbooks, just remember this: when in doubt, eat food that looks like it came from the earth, not a lab.

Good food can solve 80% of your health problems. Want to feel more energetic? Eat better. Want to think sharper? Eat better. Want to stop wondering why your jeans are plotting against you? You guessed it—eat better. Let's focus on balance, quality, and consistency. No need for kale smoothies that taste like grass or a fridge full of chia seeds you'll never touch. Small, sustainable steps will do the trick.

A Day in the Life of Healthy Living

Alright, imagine you're living your best healthy life. What does that even look like? Spoiler: it's not just endless kale and boring salads. Here's a simple breakdown to make you go, "Hey, I can do that!"

Morning:

- Hydrate: Start your day with a glass of warm water infused with lemon or ginger. It's like giving your digestive system a gentle wake-up call, not a screaming alarm.
- Move: Stretch, dance, or do yoga—whatever gets you moving. If you're really lazy, just try to touch your toes. Hey, progress is progress.
- Fuel: Breakfast is the most important meal of the day, so make it count. Think oats with nuts, eggs with avocado, or anything that makes you feel fancy and energized.

Mid-Morning:

- Snack Smart: Hungry already? No problem. Grab a handful of almonds, a piece of fruit, or Greek yogurt. Avoid the vending machine—it's not your friend.

Afternoon:

- Balanced Lunch: This is where you're the star chef of your plate. Combine protein, colorful veggies, and whole grains. Add a little healthy fat, and boom, you've got yourself a masterpiece.
- Stay Active: Take a quick walk after lunch. Call it a "digestive stroll" if it makes you feel fancy.

Evening:

- Unwind: Find a relaxing ritual that doesn't involve scrolling social media until your thumbs hurt. Meditate, journal, or just stare at a wall if that's your thing.

- Light Dinner: Keep it simple and easy to digest. Soups, salads, or grilled veggies with protein are like a bedtime story for your stomach.

Night:
- Screen-Free Time: Say goodbye to your phone an hour before bed. Yes, even TikTok. Your sleep will thank you.
- Quality Sleep: Aim for 7-8 hours of glorious, uninterrupted sleep. It's like recharging your body's Wi-Fi.

Awareness of "Don'ts"

A healthy lifestyle isn't just about adding good habits; it's equally about ditching the bad ones that derail your progress. While the dos often get all the attention, the don'ts are just as important if you want to stay on track without feeling like you're constantly backpedaling. Think of it like this: every bad habit you kick is one less hurdle on your journey to wellness. So, let's talk about some of the key "don'ts" that deserve your attention.

First up, overeating. Even the healthiest foods lose their charm when consumed in portions meant for a family of four. Sure, avocado toast is good for you, but having five slices in one sitting? Not so much. Portion control is your BFF here. It's not about depriving yourself—it's about enjoying what you eat without feeling like you need a nap afterward. Slow down, savor your food, and remember: you're eating to fuel your body, not to set a world record in competitive eating.

Then there's the sneaky culprit of sugary drinks. These bad boys are essentially liquid candy disguised as beverages. Whether it's soda, sweetened iced tea, or that fancy caramel frappuccino topped with a mountain of whipped cream, they're all loaded with sugar that your body doesn't need. Swap them for water, herbal tea, or even coffee—just skip the dessert-like additions. Your body (and your teeth) will thank you. Plus, cutting back on sugary drinks doesn't mean you can't treat yourself occasionally, but let's save that for when it's truly worth it.

Ultra-processed foods are another major "don't." If the ingredients list on the package reads like a science experiment, it's probably best to leave it on the shelf. These foods are often loaded with preservatives, artificial flavors, and a whole lot of unpronounceable stuff that does nothing for your health. Instead, stick to whole, fresh ingredients that your great-grandparents would recognize as food. The fewer steps it takes to get from farm to table, the better.

Skipping meals might seem like a fast track to weight loss, but it's more likely to land you in a vicious cycle of hunger and overindulgence. Starving yourself during the day only leads to ravenous eating later, and let's be honest—no one likes hangry you. Keep your body fueled with regular, balanced meals to maintain your energy levels and keep your metabolism running smoothly.

Finally, let's not forget mental health, which is often the most overlooked "don't." Ignoring stress or mental well-being is like inviting chaos to run your life. Stress isn't just annoying; it can wreak havoc on your body, your sleep, and your overall health. Find ways to manage it, whether that's through meditation, journaling, or even just venting to a friend. Don't let it pile up until it's unmanageable.

Ultimately, the "don'ts" are not about perfection or restriction—they're about awareness. By being mindful of these pitfalls and steering clear of them, you're setting yourself up for a lifestyle that's not only healthy but also sustainable and enjoyable. After all, wellness isn't about doing everything perfectly; it's about finding balance and making choices that genuinely make you feel good.

The Power of Quality and Quantity

In a world where Instagram influencers flaunt their perfectly arranged quinoa bowls and kale smoothies, it's easy to feel overwhelmed and confused about what "healthy eating" really means. But the truth is, it doesn't have to be that complicated. It's all about balance and remembering the golden rule: quality over quantity. The key is to choose foods that nourish your body and consume them in amounts that won't make you feel like a bear preparing for hibernation. Let's break it down.

When it comes to quality, think of it as treating your body like a temple—or at least like a rental car you don't want to return in terrible shape. Start by choosing organic and local foods whenever possible. These are the items that haven't racked up more frequent flyer miles than you this year and tend to be fresher and less processed. Seasonal foods also deserve a spotlight. Mother Nature has a way of telling you what your body needs at any given time of the year, whether it's juicy watermelon in the summer or hearty root vegetables in the winter. And let's not forget the unsung heroes of a healthy diet: healthy fats. Olive oil, nuts, and avocados are the VIPs you should invite to every meal. They not only taste great but also support your heart and brain health. Deep-fried anything, however, should remain an occasional guest, not a permanent resident.

Now, let's talk quantity, which is all about portion control and balance. Visualize your plate as a pie chart—half filled with vegetables, one-quarter with lean protein, and the last quarter with whole grains. This is the kind of math that benefits your body and doesn't require a calculator. Speaking of balance, listen to your body's cues. Eat when you're hungry, and more importantly, stop when you're full. This might sound like common sense, but it's surprisingly easy to ignore when you're binge-watching your favorite show with a bag of chips in hand. Remember, food is there to fuel you, not to act as your emotional support system. If you're sad, call a friend, journal your feelings, or even yell into a pillow — just don't try to solve your problems with an entire pint of ice cream.

Living a healthy lifestyle isn't about following every diet trend that pops up or punishing yourself for enjoying the occasional treat. It's about making small, consistent choices that prioritize both quality and quantity. Focus on foods that are good for you, enjoy them in moderation, and let go of the guilt. Life is too short to stress over every bite, but it's also too precious to ignore the importance of fueling your body with the good stuff. So, the next time you're eyeing that deep-fried brownie sundae on the menu, ask yourself: "Is this quality, quantity, or just questionable?" And then choose accordingly.

Keeping It Simple

We're not here to tell you to give up pizza forever or swear an oath to kale. A healthy lifestyle is all about balance. It's like a good rom-com — a little drama (yes, dessert counts) and a lot of happy endings. Focus on progress, not perfection, and you'll find that it's easier than you think.

Addressing Common Goals and Issues

When it comes to health, everyone's goals might look different — losing weight, gaining energy, or just surviving the day without wanting to throttle someone — but the fundamentals remain surprisingly similar. Achieving these goals doesn't require drastic measures or gimmicky diets. Instead, it's about making small, realistic changes that work for you without making you miserable. So, let's tackle some of the most common goals and issues and figure out how to handle them with a mix of practicality and just the right dash of humor.

For weight management, let's leave crash diets where they belong: in the trash. Sure, eating only celery or surviving on boiled cabbage soup for weeks might sound efficient, but it's not sustainable — and let's be honest, it's not fun either. Instead, focus on whole, nutrient-rich foods that nourish your body and keep you satisfied. A calorie deficit is important if weight loss is your goal, but it doesn't have to mean starving yourself. Eat meals that make you happy and provide energy, not ones that make you daydream about pizza while choking down plain lettuce. Remember, the goal isn't just to lose weight; it's to feel good while doing it.

If you're constantly dragging yourself out of bed and relying on caffeine as life support, boosting energy might be your top priority. Start your day with protein — eggs, Greek yogurt, or even a good smoothie can set the tone. And here's a hot take: hydration is key. Yes, water is better than coffee when it comes to energy levels (don't come for me), but coffee still has its place as the MVP of morning motivation. Just remember, balance is everything. Dehydration is a sneaky thief of energy, so keep a water bottle handy and sip often. You'll be surprised how much better you feel when your body isn't operating on a hydration deficit.

Let's talk gut health, a topic that's getting a lot of buzz lately — and for good reason. Your gut is like the ultimate party planner for your body; if it's not happy, nothing runs smoothly. Probiotics, like those found in yogurt or fermented foods, help keep the good bacteria thriving. Pair them with prebiotics, found in foods like garlic and onions, which act as fuel for your gut's bacteria squad. Together, they're the dynamic duo your digestive system needs to stay on point. So, show your gut some love and avoid overloading it with processed junk that throws the balance off.

Lastly, let's tackle stress, the sneaky saboteur of your health goals. Reducing stress doesn't mean quitting your job to live off the grid (unless that's your dream, in which case, go for it). Sometimes, it's as simple as taking a few deep breaths, meditating for five minutes, or even having a good scream into a pillow when life feels overwhelming. Do whatever helps you unwind, and don't underestimate the power of laughter, good company, or just zoning out with your favorite Netflix show.

Remember, health isn't about perfection. It's about finding what works for you and sticking with it. Small steps lead to big changes, so tackle your goals with patience, humor, and a generous dose of self-compassion.

A Holistic Approach

Health isn't just about food and exercise. It's about feeling good mentally, emotionally, and socially. Surround yourself with people who make you laugh, find hobbies that bring you joy, and never underestimate the power of a good nap.

Sustainability Is Key

Sustainability isn't just for the planet; it's for your habits too. Extreme diets and insane workout regimens might look cool on Instagram, but they're like wearing heels to a marathon—not practical. Instead, aim for small changes that add up over time.

- Meal Prep: A little planning goes a long way in avoiding pizza delivery every other day.
- Stay Accountable: Find a buddy who'll remind you to eat a salad now and then.
- Celebrate Small Wins: Drank enough water today? That's a win. Did a 10-minute workout? Another win. Treat yourself (but maybe not with cake).

Adopting a healthy lifestyle is like learning a dance. At first, it's awkward, but with practice, it becomes second nature. Remember, it's not about being perfect; it's about showing up for yourself. Keep it simple, keep it fun, and keep going. Because at the end of the day, your health is your most loyal partner in life. Treat it right, and it'll have your back every step of the way.

Morning Routine: Setting the Tone for a Healthier Day

Your morning sets the tone for the rest of your day. While it's tempting to reach for your phone first thing, scroll through notifications, and dive into the chaos of life, there's a better way to start. A mindful, intentional morning routine can significantly improve your mental and physical well-being. Let's break it down step-by-step—because waking up healthy and happy shouldn't feel like rocket science.

The Power of Waking Up Mindfully

Mornings are like Mondays—nobody really loves them, but they keep coming. Instead of starting your day by doom-scrolling through memes and emails, let's talk about how to wake up like a boss. Spoiler alert: it doesn't involve hitting snooze five times or sleeping until your alarm starts questioning your life choices. It's all about waking up mindfully and making those first minutes count.

Step 1: Wake Up and Breathe (Seriously, Just Breathe)

Congratulations, you've survived another night! Before you grab your phone and start panicking about the 500 unread messages, take a moment to *just breathe*. It's free, it's simple, and unlike most life advice, it actually works.

Enter Jose Silva's Method. This fancy-sounding technique is basically like giving your brain a pep talk before it officially clocks in. Close your eyes (don't fall back asleep!), visualize something that makes you happy, and set some positive intentions. Think,

"Today, I will crush it," not, "Today, I will avoid eye contact with my boss."

Next, let's talk about deep breathing. Sure, you've been breathing your whole life, but have you been doing it right? Try this: inhale for 4 seconds, hold for 7 seconds, and exhale for 8 seconds. It's like a spa day for your lungs. Not only will this calm your racing mind, but it'll also energize you faster than your first sip of coffee (well, almost). Plus, it's way cheaper than therapy.

Step 2: Affirmations and Gratitude (Channel Your Inner Optimist)

Affirmations may sound like something out of a self-help seminar, but don't knock it till you try it. They're like personal pep talks. Look in the mirror (or imagine yourself looking amazing) and say something like, "I am capable," "I am strong," or "I will not lose my temper in traffic today." Bonus points if you don't roll your eyes halfway through.

Pair this with a little gratitude journaling. Grab a notebook or just mentally list three things you're grateful for. It can be big things like your health or small wins like the fact that your favorite cereal was on sale. Gratitude shifts your focus from "Ugh, why is it morning again?" to "Wow, I'm kind of winning at life."

Step 3: Stretch It Out (Without Feeling Like a Gym Class Dropout)

Stretching in the morning is like hitting the "refresh" button on your body. You've been lying still all night (unless you're a ninja in your sleep), and your muscles deserve a little TLC.

Start with easy stretches that don't require Olympic-level flexibility. While still in bed, try a big full-body stretch, reaching your arms above your head and pointing your toes like you're auditioning for Swan Lake. Then roll out of bed and touch your toes (or your knees—no judgment).

Not only does stretching wake up your body, but it also reduces stiffness, improves circulation, and makes you feel slightly more human. Think of it as the pregame before you take on the day.

Starting your morning mindfully isn't rocket science—it's just about slowing down, breathing, and treating yourself with a little kindness. No complicated gadgets or overpriced routines required. So, the next time your alarm rings, ditch the panic and start your day like the mindful rockstar you are. You've got this!

Nourish Your Body First: Starting with Fats

Let's get one thing straight: fats aren't the villain in your health story. In fact, they're the unsung heroes—like the quirky sidekick in a rom-com who ends up saving the day. And when it comes to starting your morning right, a spoonful of healthy fat can do wonders. No, this isn't about frying bacon or dipping a croissant in butter (though we've all been tempted). This is about smart fats. Specifically, ghee.

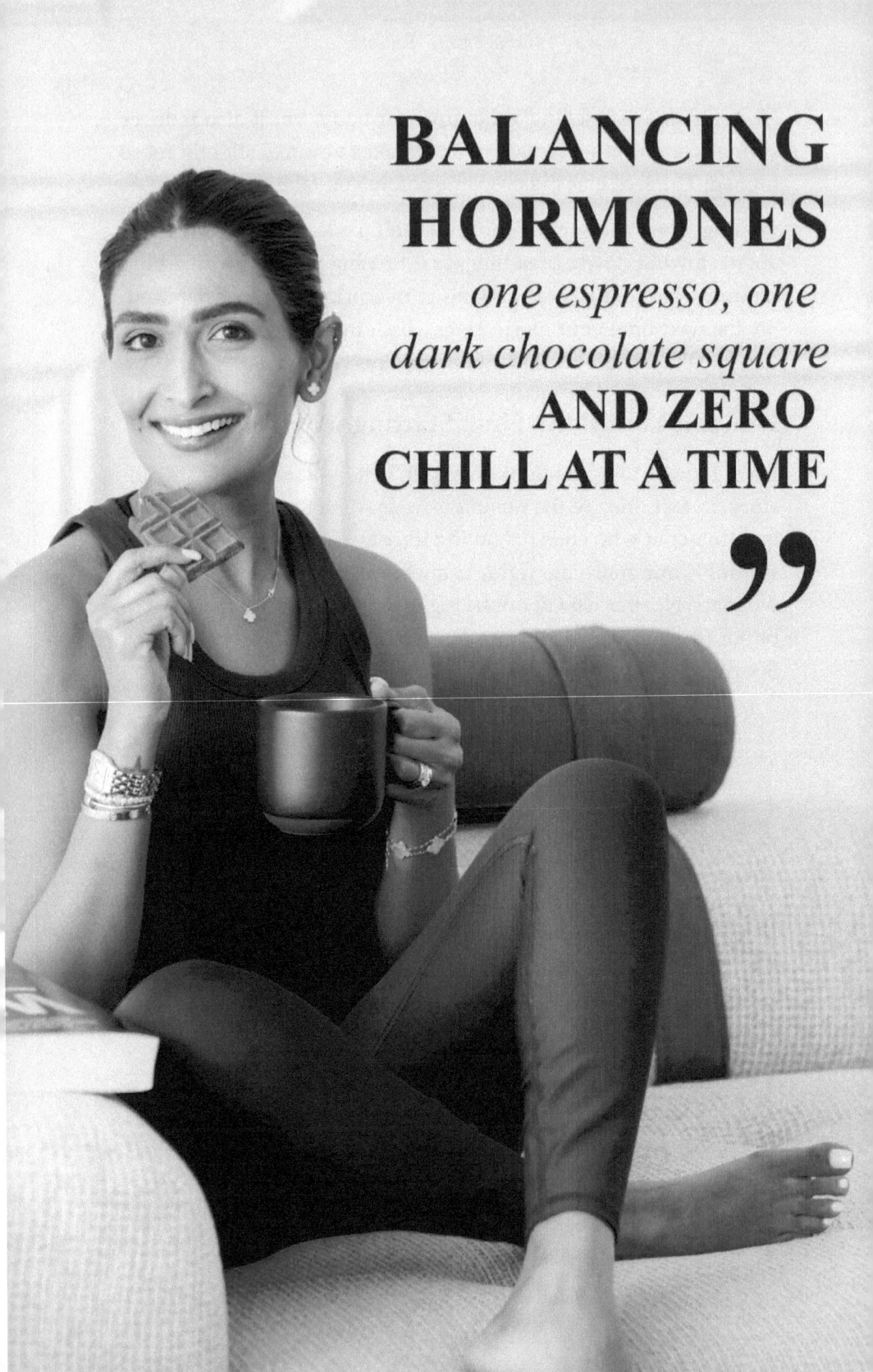

Why Ghee Deserves a Spot in Your Morning Routine

Picture this: it's 7 AM, and you're trying to convince yourself that life is worth waking up for. Enter ghee, that golden, velvety, superhero-in-a-spoon. A tablespoon of this clarified butter doesn't just taste luxurious—it kickstarts your day like a motivational TED Talk for your insides.

- *Boosts Digestion:* Ghee is like that friend who comes over and cleans up your messy apartment. It supports digestion by lubricating your gut and encouraging smooth digestion (pun intended). So, if you've been feeling like your stomach's been running on dial-up, ghee is here to upgrade you to high-speed fiber-optic health.
- *Sustainable Energy*: Unlike your caffeine crash or sugar coma, ghee offers slow-burning energy. It's like turning on your car and realizing the tank is full (a rare and beautiful moment). With ghee, you won't be raiding the snack drawer at 10 AM like a stressed-out squirrel.
- *Hormonal Harmony:* Ghee is rich in fat-soluble vitamins like A, D, E, and K, which are essential for hormonal balance. It's like giving your body a much-needed pep talk: "Let's keep the hormones chill today, alright?"

Not a Fan of Ghee? No Problem.

If ghee feels a little too traditional for your modern palate, there are plenty of alternatives that don't skimp on benefits.

- *Coconut Oil:* Tropical and versatile, this oil is perfect for plant-based enthusiasts. Bonus: it makes you feel fancy, like you're vacationing in the Maldives.
- *Olive Oil:* Your Mediterranean go-to. Not ideal for coffee (don't try it, seriously), but great for savory breakfasts.
- *Avocado:* Yes, millennials, this is your moment. Mash it, slice it, or blend it—avocado is the Beyoncé of breakfast fats.

Why Fats First Thing in the Morning?

Let's break it down. When you start your day with healthy fats, your body feels nourished, not overloaded. It kickstarts your metabolism, sharpens your brain, and gives your body the building blocks it needs to thrive. Plus, it's a great way to tell your stomach, "Relax, we're eating grown-up food now."

Healthy fats also stabilize blood sugar levels, which means fewer mood swings and less temptation to throw your coffee mug at someone by 9 AM. Your brain gets a boost too—it's made up of 60% fat, after all—so a morning dose of ghee or its alternatives is like feeding your brain the equivalent of high-octane fuel.

Starting your day with fats is like giving your body a standing ovation before it even gets out of bed. Whether it's ghee, coconut oil, or avocado, adding healthy fats to your morning sets the tone for a day of balance and energy. So, grab that spoon and toast to your health—just maybe don't try spreading ghee on toast. Save that for your paratha.

Turmeric-Ginger Tea or Shot: The Morning Potion You Didn't Know You Needed

Let's face it: mornings can be rough. Your alarm clock goes off like a personal attack, and your brain is still buffering. Enter the turmeric-ginger tea or shot—a morning elixir so powerful, it might as well come with a cape. This golden-hued potion isn't just trendy; it's like hiring a superhero squad for your body. Anti-inflammatory powers? Check. Immunity boost? Check. A gentle wake-up call for your digestive system? Double-check.

Turmeric, ginger, and black pepper are like the ultimate wellness trio, bringing centuries of ancient medicinal wisdom into your cup. They don't just add flavor to your food—they can also support your body in ways that make you feel unstoppable (or at least much better).

Turmeric: This vibrant yellow spice is famous for its active compound, curcumin, which is packed with powerful anti-inflammatory and antioxidant properties. It helps:

- Reduce inflammation, making it great for soothing joint pain and muscle aches.
- Support brain health by protecting against oxidative stress.
- Aid digestion and promote gut health.

Ginger: Ginger is more than just a zingy spice—it's a digestive and immune-boosting hero. It helps:

- Calm nausea and bloating by promoting healthy digestion.
- Strengthen the immune system with its antibacterial and antiviral properties.
- Relieve pain and muscle soreness, especially after workouts or long days.

Black Pepper: You might not think much of black pepper, but it's the secret ingredient that makes turmeric even more effective. It contains piperine, a compound that:

- Increases curcumin absorption by up to 2,000%, ensuring your body gets all the benefits.
- Enhances digestion and metabolism.
- Has its own anti-inflammatory and antioxidant properties.

Why You Need This Trio in Your Life

Together, turmeric, ginger, and black pepper create a powerhouse elixir that fights inflammation, supports digestion, boosts immunity, and keeps you feeling your best. So, the next time you sip on this golden drink, know that you're fueling your body with nature's best medicine!

How to Make Your Morning Magic

The beauty of turmeric-ginger tea or shots is that they're as simple or fancy as you want them to be. No need to overcomplicate it—this isn't a Michelin-star recipe.

The Simple Shot (With a Power Boost!)

1. Grate a small chunk of fresh ginger and fresh turmeric (or use powdered versions if you're in a rush).
2. Add the juice of half a lemon, a drizzle of honey, and a splash of water.
3. Don't forget black pepper! A pinch enhances turmeric absorption, making the shot even more effective.
4. Stir well and shoot it back like a tequila shot—except this one leaves you energized, not regretting last night's choices.

Make-Ahead Options for Convenience

Option 1: Paste (Store for 1 Week in the Fridge)

1. Blend ½ cup grated ginger, ½ cup grated turmeric, ½ tsp black pepper, and the juice of 2 lemons into a smooth paste.
2. Store in an airtight glass jar in the fridge.
3. How to use: Take ½ teaspoon of the paste, mix it with warm water, honey, and a little more lemon for a quick shot every morning.

Option 2: Frozen Cubes (Store for 2-3 Weeks)

1. Blend ginger, turmeric, black pepper, lemon juice, and honey with a little water into a smooth mixture.
2. Pour into ice cube trays and freeze.
3. How to use: Drop a cube into warm water or tea, stir, and sip! You can also blend it into smoothies for an immunity boost.

Tea for the Soul

- Boil water and add fresh ginger slices and a teaspoon of turmeric.
- Simmer for 5-10 minutes, then strain into a mug.
- Add a pinch of black pepper (it helps your body absorb curcumin) and a touch of honey for sweetness. Bonus points for a cinnamon stick—it's like giving your tea a warm hug.

Feeling adventurous? Try adding a sprinkle of cinnamon for natural sweetness and balanced blood sugar, or a dash of cayenne for a fiery metabolism boost. And let's not forget black pepper—it's not just for flavor; it supercharges turmeric's benefits by increasing absorption.

Want to take things up a notch? Add a splash of coconut milk for a creamy, latte-like vibe.

Before turmeric lattes became a trendy café staple, our grandmothers were already making this golden elixir—Haldi Ka Doodh—for generations. It's been the go-to remedy for colds, joint pain, and overall well-being.

How to Make It:

1. Warm a cup of milk (dairy or plant-based).
2. Add ½ teaspoon turmeric, a pinch of black pepper, and ¼ teaspoon cinnamon (great for blood sugar balance and a cozy flavor).
3. Stir in a teaspoon of honey for natural sweetness.
4. Optional: Add a dash of ginger powder or cardamom for extra warmth.
5. Simmer for a few minutes, pour into your favorite mug, and enjoy!

Starting your day with a turmeric-ginger tea, shot, or latte is like giving your body a pep talk: "You've got this." It's quick, easy, and packed with health benefits.

So next time you're tempted to skip breakfast or dive straight into caffeine chaos, sip on this golden goodness instead. Your immune system (and digestive tract) will thank you. Plus, who doesn't love starting the day feeling like a wellness influencer?

Gut Cleanse with Morning Hydration

Before you dive into your day like a caffeinated squirrel, let's talk about the *real* MVP of your morning routine: hydration. Your gut has been working overtime all night, and it deserves a little love. Morning hydration is like a fresh reboot for your digestive system—a "good morning" text for your body. Whether it's lemon water, fennel water, or fenugreek water, these liquid heroes are here to cleanse, balance, and get your gut grooving.

Your body is basically a sponge after eight hours of sleep. When you wake up, your cells are parched and your gut is ready to detox. Hydrating first thing in the morning jump-starts your metabolism, flushes out toxins, and gives your digestive system a friendly nudge. Plus, it sets the tone for healthier choices throughout the day (because who wants to ruin that detox glow with a sugary pastry?).

Lemon Water: The Classic Detox Darling

Lemon water is the Beyoncé of morning drinks—always in the spotlight and with good reason. A squeeze of lemon in warm water is the simplest way to wake up your digestive system.

- Detoxification Support: Lemon water acts like a natural plumber, flushing out toxins and keeping things moving.

- Alkalizing Effect: Despite being acidic, lemons help balance your body's pH, creating an environment your gut bacteria will throw a party for.
- Vitamin C Boost: It gives your immune system a gentle "you got this" boost, perfect for tackling the day ahead.

Pro tip: Sip it warm and imagine you're at a spa (even if you're actually just sitting in your kitchen in mismatched socks).

Fennel (Saunf) Water: The Digestive Whisperer

If lemon water is Beyoncé, fennel water is the quiet genius who knows all the answers but doesn't show off. Fennel seeds, soaked overnight and sipped in the morning, are a godsend for your gut.

- Aids Digestion: Fennel water soothes your stomach like a lullaby for your gut lining. Say goodbye to bloating and gas.
- Reduces Cravings: Its mildly sweet taste helps curb those mid-morning snack attacks.
- Rich in Antioxidants: Fennel seeds are packed with compounds that keep your gut happy and inflammation at bay.

Bonus: You'll feel like you're channeling some ancient Ayurvedic wisdom.

Fenugreek (Methi) Water: The Hormone Whisperer

For the overachievers out there, fenugreek water is like having a personal assistant for your hormones and blood sugar levels. Soak the seeds overnight, and your body will thank you.

- Blood Sugar Control: Methi water helps stabilize your glucose levels, making it a great choice for anyone prone to sugar crashes.
- Hormonal Balance: Fenugreek works behind the scenes to support your body's endocrine system, which is a fancy way of saying it helps keep things running smoothly.

- Digestive Health: It encourages smooth digestion, so your gut doesn't feel like it's hosting a wrestling match.

Whether you choose lemon, fennel, or fenugreek water, the goal is the same: a gut that's ready to take on the world (or at least your breakfast). Mix it up depending on your mood or health goals, and remember: hydration is your gut's love language.

Gut Cleanse Smoothie: The Ultimate Breakfast Hug for Your Belly

Let's face it—your gut has been through a lot. Late-night snacks, questionable takeout, and that extra cheese pizza you swore you wouldn't finish. But mornings are a chance to make amends, and a gut cleanse smoothie is basically a heartfelt apology in a glass. Packed with fiber, hydration, and a whole lot of green goodness, it's your gut's BFF, ready to set things right.

Think of your gut as the unsung hero of your body—quietly working behind the scenes to keep you energized, happy, and bloating-free. A high-fiber smoothie not only helps cleanse your digestive system but also gives it the hydration it craves after a long night of hard work (because yes, even your gut deserves a break).

Fiber is like the Marie Kondo of your digestive system, tidying up everything that doesn't spark joy (or health). Pair it with some water-rich ingredients, and you've got a refreshing, nutrient-packed breakfast that screams, "I've got my life together!" (even if you really don't).

The Recipe: The Ultimate Gut-Cleanse Smoothie

- 200ml Coconut Water: A hydrating base loaded with electrolytes to keep your digestion smooth and your body refreshed.

- **4 to 5 Cubes Pineapple:** Naturally sweet and packed with bromelain, an enzyme that aids digestion and reduces bloating.
- **2 Celery Stalks:** A powerhouse of fiber and antioxidants, promoting gut health and hydration.
- **1 Pc Ginger:** Known for its anti-inflammatory and digestive benefits, ginger soothes the stomach and supports digestion.
- **1 Pc Turmeric or 1 Tsp Powder:** A golden superfood with powerful anti-inflammatory and detoxifying properties.
- **7 to 8 Slices Cucumber:** Refreshing, hydrating, and gentle on the stomach.
- **1/2 Lime:** Adds a tangy freshness while supporting digestion and detoxification.

Optional extras: If you like a little extra spice, add a pinch of black pepper to enhance turmeric absorption!

How to Make It

Blend everything together until it's as smooth as your best pickup line. Pour it into your favorite glass or mason jar (because aesthetics matter), and sip it slowly. Bonus points if you enjoy it while sitting in sunlight, pretending you're on a wellness retreat.

Why This Smoothie Works

Fiber is the secret weapon your gut didn't know it needed. It helps move things along (you know what we mean) and feeds the good bacteria in your gut. Think of it as throwing a little party for your microbiome.

Hydration is equally crucial. After a night of zero water intake, your body needs a big gulp of liquid love. The water-rich ingredients in this smoothie work together to refresh your system and keep you glowing from the inside out.

High-Fiber, High-Protein Breakfast: Fuel for Champions (and Regular Humans)

Breakfast is the Beyoncé of meals — it sets the tone for the day. Skip it, and you'll be hangry by 11 a.m., eating chips in shame. But nail it? You'll be out there solving problems, making deals, and probably looking fabulous while doing it. The secret? A high-fiber, high-protein breakfast that keeps you full, focused, and far away from the vending machine.

Fiber and protein are like the ultimate power couple. Fiber keeps your digestion smooth (no awkward mid-meeting tummy growls), and protein fuels your energy reserves like a steady IV of motivation. Together, they're the breakfast duo you didn't know you needed, offering long-lasting energy without the sugar crash.

Non-Vegetarian Options: Keep It Eggcellent

Eggs are the OG breakfast MVP. They are packed with high-quality protein, vitamins, and essential minerals. Whether boiled, scrambled, or turned into a Michelin-worthy omelet, eggs are a versatile powerhouse.

1. Classic Scrambled Eggs with Whole Wheat Toast: Lightly scrambled eggs cooked with a touch of olive oil, garlic, and spinach served on toasted whole-wheat bread provide the perfect balance of protein and fiber. Add a side of avocado for healthy fats.

2. Omelet with a Twist: Ditch the boring omelet and go for a fully loaded version with bell peppers, mushrooms, spinach, and a sprinkle of feta cheese. Pair it with a bowl of Greek yogurt for an extra protein punch.

3. Chicken Breakfast Wrap: Shred some leftover grilled chicken and wrap it in a whole wheat or multigrain tortilla with lettuce, tomatoes, and a light yogurt dressing.

4. Smoked Salmon and Avocado Toast: A slice of sourdough topped with avocado mash, smoked salmon, and a poached egg is a nutrient-dense, high-protein breakfast rich in Omega-3s.

5. Egg and Quinoa Bowl: Pair boiled eggs with cooked quinoa, roasted cherry tomatoes, and a drizzle of lemon juice for a well-balanced meal packed with fiber and protein.

Vegetarian/Vegan Options: No Eggs, No Problem

Who says a protein-packed meal needs eggs? Whether you're vegan, allergic, or just looking to switch things up, there are plenty of nourishing and satisfying options to keep you energized. From savory pancakes to creamy chia pudding, these wholesome recipes prove that plant-based eating can be both easy and delicious.

6. Lentil-Based Pancakes (Dal Chilla): Dal chillas are high in protein, easy to make, and taste like a hug on a plate. Serve with chutneys or Greek yogurt for extra nutrition.

7. Protein-Packed Oatmeal: Cook oats with almond or coconut milk, then pile on toppings like nuts, seeds, and fresh fruit. Add a drizzle of nut butter for extra protein.

8. Tofu Scramble: For a vegan twist on scrambled eggs, crumble tofu and cook it with turmeric, black salt (for an eggy flavor), and bell peppers.

9. Chia Seed Pudding: Soak chia seeds in almond milk overnight, then top with fruits, nuts, and granola for a no-fuss, protein-rich breakfast.

10. Quinoa and Chickpea Salad: Combine cooked quinoa with chickpeas, cucumbers, tomatoes, and a lemon-tahini dressing for a refreshing and filling meal.

South Indian Staples: Fermented, Flavorful, and Fantastic

South Indian breakfasts are a masterclass in gut-friendly, fiber-rich meals. Rooted in centuries-old traditions, these dishes not only tantalize the taste buds but also nourish the body with essential nutrients. Packed with probiotics, fiber, and plant-based protein, these wholesome meals promote digestion, sustain energy levels, and keep you feeling full longer.

11. Idli with Sambar: Fermented rice and urad dal idlis served with protein-rich sambar make for a delicious, gut-friendly meal.

12. Pesarattu (Green Moong Dal Dosa): A crispy dosa made with green gram dal is rich in protein and pairs well with ginger chutney.

13. Ragi Dosa with Coconut Chutney: A nutritious, gluten-free dosa made with ragi (finger millet) flour is a fiber powerhouse.

14. Millet Upma: Swap traditional semolina with millets like foxtail or barnyard millet for a protein-packed, fiber-rich breakfast.

15. Avarekalu Akki Roti (Hyacinth Bean Flatbread): A Karnataka favorite, this protein-rich roti made from rice flour and hyacinth beans is both nourishing and tasty.

North Indian Delights: Hearty and Wholesome

North Indian cuisine is a treasure trove of flavors, offering a perfect balance of taste and nutrition. From protein-packed dishes to fiber-rich flatbreads, these wholesome meals are not only satisfying but also nourishing. Whether you're looking for a hearty breakfast or a light yet fulfilling meal, these traditional recipes bring the best of North Indian flavors to your plate.

16. Paneer Bhurji with Multigrain Roti: Scrambled cottage cheese cooked with onions, tomatoes, and spices makes a high-protein, delicious breakfast.

17. Sprouts Chaat: Sprouted moong, chana, and black gram tossed with onions, tomatoes, and lemon juice create a protein-packed chaat.

18. Missi Roti with Raita: This high-protein, fiber-rich flatbread made from besan (chickpea flour) pairs perfectly with cucumber raita.

19. Bajra Khichdi: Made with bajra (pearl millet) and lentils, this hearty dish is perfect for a nutrient-dense breakfast.

20. Methi Thepla with Yogurt: A Gujarati favorite, fenugreek (methi) leaves mixed with whole wheat flour make a fiber-rich flatbread that pairs well with probiotic-rich yogurt.

Continental Picks: A Touch of Global Goodness

Start your day with flavors from around the world! Whether you crave something light and refreshing or rich and satisfying, these continental-inspired breakfasts bring the perfect balance of taste and nutrition. Packed with fiber, protein, and healthy fats, each dish offers a wholesome way to fuel your morning with global goodness.

21. Avocado Toast on Sourdough: Topped with cherry tomatoes, feta, and a poached egg, this meal offers fiber, protein, and healthy fats.

22. Smoothie Bowl: Blend bananas, berries, Greek yogurt (or plant-based alternatives), and a handful of nuts for a refreshing breakfast.

23. Overnight Oats: Oats soaked overnight in almond milk with chia seeds, topped with nuts and fruits, provide a balanced, fiber-rich meal.

24. Nut Butter and Banana Toast: A slice of multigrain toast with almond or peanut butter and banana slices makes for a satisfying, protein-packed start to the day.

25. Cottage Cheese and Fruit Bowl: A bowl of fresh cottage cheese with diced mangoes, strawberries, and a drizzle of honey offers a protein boost.

Gluten-Free Goodness: Because Everyone Deserves a Great Breakfast

Starting your day with a nourishing meal is essential, but finding gluten-free options that are both delicious and satisfying can be a challenge. Whether you're avoiding gluten for health reasons or simply exploring new flavors, these wholesome breakfast ideas are packed with nutrients, flavor, and variety. From warm porridges to savory pancakes and protein-rich alternatives, these recipes ensure that you never have to compromise on taste or nutrition.

26. Millet Porridge: Bajra or ragi porridge cooked with coconut milk and naturally sweetened with dates makes for a nutritious meal.

27. Besan Chilla: Savory pancakes made from chickpea flour, loaded with veggies, and served with mint chutney.

28. Quinoa Upma: A high-protein version of upma made with quinoa instead of semolina.

29. Sweet Potato Hash: Cubed sweet potatoes stir-fried with bell peppers and tofu make a hearty meal.

30. Almond Flour Pancakes: A fluffy, protein-rich alternative to regular pancakes made using almond flour and eggs (or flax eggs for a vegan version).

Why This Works

This breakfast combo is your ticket to sustained energy, fewer snack cravings, and the smug satisfaction of knowing you ate something nutritious. It's balanced, delicious, and won't leave you slumped over your desk by 2 p.m. Breakfast doesn't have to be boring or a chore. Think of it as a little gift to yourself, a moment to start your day with intention — and a whole lot of yum.

Fruits and Nuts: The MVPs of a Balanced Breakfast

Let's talk fruits and nuts — nature's snack-sized, nutrient-packed powerhouses. They're the OG superfoods, predating every trendy health bar, and they don't even need flashy packaging. But before you go throwing a fruit salad into a mixing bowl or eating almonds like popcorn, let's get into the *how, when,* and *why* of this dynamic duo.

Timing is Everything

Think of fruits and nuts as supporting characters, not the main event of your breakfast. The best time to enjoy them? Mid-morning or alongside breakfast. Why? Fruits contain natural sugars, and eaten solo, they can spike your blood sugar faster than you can say "banana." Pair them with nuts, and voilà — instant balance. The fats and protein in nuts slow down sugar absorption, giving you steady energy rather than a rollercoaster ride of hunger pangs.

Portion Control: Because More Isn't Always Better

Here's the thing about fruits: they're sweet, juicy, and deceptively innocent-looking. But too much of a good thing can turn your breakfast into a sugar bomb. Stick to a portion — think one medium-sized fruit or a cup of berries.

Nuts, on the other hand, are like that friend who's fun but a little too extra in large doses. A small handful (around 10-12 almonds or walnuts) is all you need to keep the party in your stomach going strong. Remember, they're high in good fats, but even good fats come with calories attached.

Balance is Key

The secret to a perfect fruit-and-nut combo lies in pairing. Combine fruits with a handful of nuts or seeds to create a satisfying, nutrient-dense snack. For example:

- Apples and walnuts: Crunchy, sweet, and a brain-boosting duo.
- Berries and almonds: A pop of flavor with a side of protein.
- Papaya and chia seeds: Tropical vibes with a fiber kick.

Not only does this combo keep you full for longer, but it also improves nutrient absorption. Think of it like teamwork: the healthy fats in nuts help your body better absorb the vitamins from fruits.

Suggestions Based on Diet Type

If your breakfast leans heavily on protein (think eggs or oats), pair it with light, refreshing fruits like apples, berries, or a slice of papaya. These fruits complement protein without feeling overwhelming.

Need an energy boost? Enter nuts like soaked almonds, cashews, or even a sprinkle of chia seeds on your yogurt or smoothie bowl. Soaked almonds, in particular, are a crowd favorite — they're easier to digest and feel oddly fancy.

The Why of It All

Fruits and nuts aren't just about taste — they're about function. Fruits provide essential vitamins, antioxidants, and hydration, while nuts bring healthy fats, protein, and that satisfying crunch.

Together, they're like the ultimate breakfast dream team, making sure you're energized, satisfied, and ready to conquer the day.

Bread: The Staple Superstar

Ah, bread. It's the reliable bestie of breakfast — a culinary blank canvas waiting to be transformed into a masterpiece. Whether it's slathered with butter, toasted to perfection, or used as the base for an open-faced sandwich, bread has earned its place as a morning staple. But before you grab just any loaf, let's chat about the dos and don'ts of bread in the morning. Because, like life, not all bread is created equal.

For many, bread is more than just food — it's a source of comfort. From childhood PB&J sandwiches to the warm, buttered toast that accompanies a cozy breakfast, bread is deeply tied to emotions and nostalgia. This emotional dependency often leads people to reach for the quickest, most convenient option, typically refined white bread. However, not all bread provides the same nutritional value, and making a mindful choice can transform your morning routine from sluggish to energized.

Many of us opt for quick fixes — pre-packaged loaves that are high in refined flour and preservatives. While these are convenient, they often lack the fiber, protein, and healthy fats needed for sustained energy. Instead of reaching for ultra-processed bread, why not explore options that nourish the body and mind?

The Emotional Connection: Why We Crave Bread

Bread is one of those foods that triggers nostalgia. The scent of freshly baked bread can transport us back to childhood, to comforting meals with family, or even remind us of travel experiences. This emotional connection is powerful and explains why many people find it difficult to cut bread from their diet, even when trying to make healthier choices.

But here's the thing—enjoying bread doesn't mean sacrificing nutrition. The key lies in choosing the right kind of bread. When we make conscious choices, we can turn this staple into a source of nourishment rather than just a quick fix for hunger.

Gluten-Free Options: Because Bread Shouldn't Judge

If gluten isn't your thing (whether by choice or because your gut said, "Nope"), there are plenty of alternatives. Gone are the days of sad, crumbly gluten-free loaves that taste like cardboard. Now, you've got:

- **Millet Bread**: Naturally gluten-free, packed with nutrients, and has a mildly sweet, nutty flavor.
- **Buckwheat Bread**: Despite the name, buckwheat is gluten-free and full of fiber, making it a hearty and delicious choice.
- **Brown Rice Bread**: A mild-tasting, easy-to-digest option for those avoiding wheat.
- **Sourdough (Yes, Really!)**: Traditional sourdough, if made from gluten-free grains or properly fermented wheat, can be tolerated by some people with mild gluten sensitivities.

SOURDOUGH:
proof that good
things rise
with patience,
wild yeast,
and a whole
lot of carbs

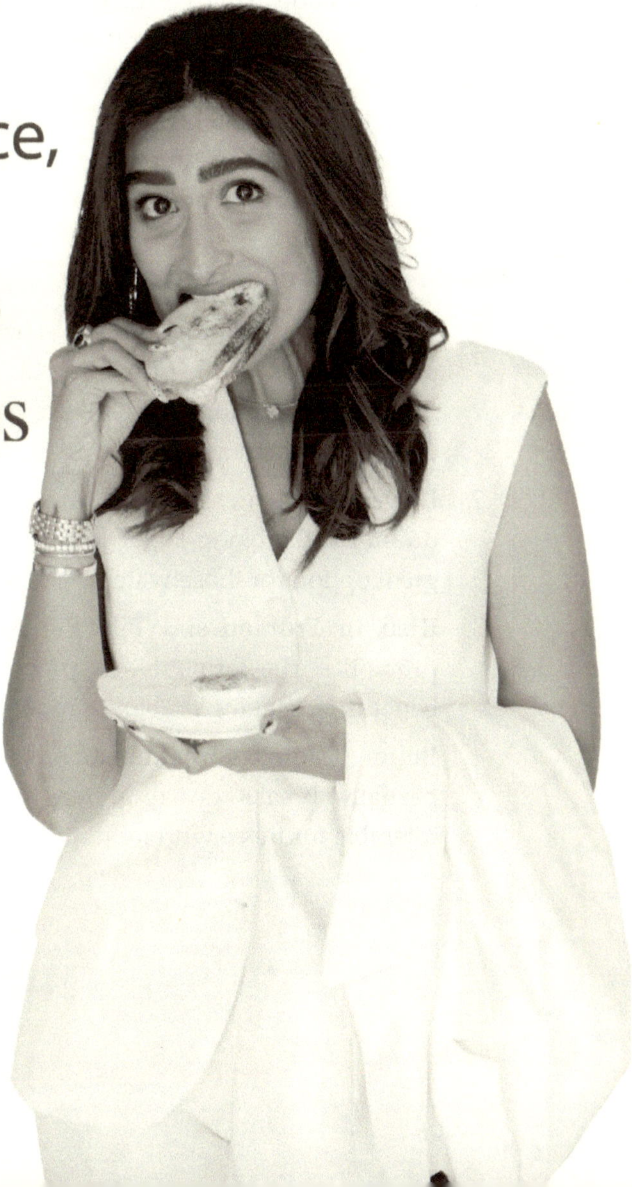

Sourdough: The Trend That's Here to Stay

If there's one bread that has taken the world by storm recently, it's sourdough. Walk into any artisanal bakery, and you'll see beautifully crusty loaves, often with a signature scoring pattern on top. But what makes sourdough so special, and why is it a better choice than most commercially available breads?

The Science Behind Sourdough

Sourdough is made using a fermentation process that relies on wild yeast and lactic acid bacteria rather than commercial yeast. This process gives sourdough its distinct tangy flavor and chewy texture. Unlike standard bread, which rises quickly due to added yeast, sourdough takes time to develop—sometimes up to 48 hours—resulting in a bread that's easier to digest.

Health Benefits of Sourdough

1. **Gut-Friendly Fermentation**: The natural fermentation process helps break down phytic acid, which can inhibit nutrient absorption. This makes sourdough easier on the digestive system and more nutrient-dense.
2. **Lower Glycemic Index**: Unlike white bread, sourdough doesn't spike blood sugar levels as drastically, making it a great option for those watching their blood sugar.
3. **Rich in Probiotics**: While the baking process kills live probiotics, the fermentation process still offers gut health benefits by making prebiotics more available.
4. **Better Gluten Breakdown**: The fermentation process partially breaks down gluten, making sourdough more tolerable for those with mild gluten sensitivities.

Pairing Ideas: Making Bread Fancy

Bread by itself is fine, but why settle for fine when you can have fabulous? Here are a few ways to turn your toast into a morning showstopper:

1. **Avocado Toast with a Kick**: Spread a ripe avocado onto your bread, sprinkle chili flakes, and maybe add a drizzle of olive oil or a poached egg. It's healthy, Instagrammable, and tastes like a little slice of heaven.

2. **Nut Butter and Banana Slices**: Grab your favorite nut butter (just make sure it's the no-added-sugar kind), spread generously, and top with banana slices. Add a sprinkle of cinnamon for extra flair. Pro tip: Almond butter on sourdough is a match made in breakfast heaven.

3. **Hummus and Veggies**: Smear on some hummus and layer with cucumber, tomato, or even roasted red peppers. It's like a mini salad on toast, and who doesn't love multitasking?

4. **Classic Jam (with a Twist)**: Use whole-fruit jam or mash some fresh berries for a DIY topping. Pair it with nut butter for that iconic sweet-salty combo.

5. **Egg and Greens on Toast**: Scramble some eggs with spinach, kale, or arugula and pile them onto a thick slice of sourdough. This combination provides protein, healthy fats, and fiber, keeping you full for hours.

Easy and Quick Breakfasts with Bread

Mornings can be hectic, but that doesn't mean breakfast has to be skipped. Here are some easy, healthy, and quick bread-based breakfasts:

- **Overnight Bread Pudding**: Cube whole-grain bread, soak it in almond milk and cinnamon overnight, and bake it in the morning.

- **French Toast with a Healthy Twist**: Use whole-grain or sourdough bread and swap out refined sugar for maple syrup or honey.
- **Egg-in-a-Hole**: Cut a hole in a slice of sourdough, drop an egg in, and cook until crispy.
- **Breakfast Sandwich**: Whole-grain bread, avocado, turkey, and spinach—simple, nutritious, and filling.

Bread is more than just a meal staple—it's an experience, a comfort, and a source of nourishment when chosen wisely. Whether you're opting for a hearty whole-grain loaf, experimenting with gluten-free alternatives, or embracing the sourdough trend, the key is to be mindful of your choices. Avoid highly processed, sugar-laden bread, and instead go for options that fuel your body and mind.

So the next time you reach for bread in the morning, think beyond just filling your stomach. Think about how it can be a delicious, nutrient-dense part of your day—because breakfast is too important to settle for anything less.

The Science Behind Morning Habits

So, what's the deal with all these morning food rituals? Is it just a trend, or is there actual science behind it? Spoiler alert: It's the latter. Let's break down how these habits work their magic.

- *Improved Digestion*

Starting your day with fiber-rich foods like whole-grain bread, millet bread, or sourdough helps keep your digestive system in check. Fiber acts like a broom for your gut, sweeping away toxins and keeping things running smoothly. Combine that with hydration (hello, lemon water or fennel tea), and you're setting the stage for a gut that's happy and healthy.

- *Regulated Blood Sugar*

Ever had a sugary breakfast and found yourself starving an hour later? That's your blood sugar doing the cha-cha. High-carb, low-protein foods cause spikes and crashes that leave you feeling hangry and sluggish. Adding protein and healthy fats to your bread — like avocado or nut butter — slows down digestion, keeping your blood sugar stable and your mood intact.

- *Boosted Energy Levels*

Carbs often get a bad rap, but the right ones (looking at you, whole-grain bread) are your body's preferred energy source. Pair them with nutrient-dense toppings, and you've got a breakfast that fuels you for hours. It's like turning your body into a well-oiled machine instead of one running on fumes.

- *Enhanced Mood*

Believe it or not, what you eat in the morning can impact your mood. Foods rich in healthy fats (avocado, nuts) and complex carbs (whole grains) help produce serotonin, the "feel-good" hormone. Meanwhile, avoiding sugar crashes means you're less likely to snap at your coworker for breathing too loudly.

Elevating Your Mornings, Elevating Your Life

The way we begin our mornings sets the rhythm for the entire day. While it's easy to fall into the trap of rushing through the first few hours, mindlessly scrolling through notifications, or skipping essential self-care, a structured and mindful routine can bring immense benefits to both body and mind. As explored throughout this discussion, embracing morning rituals that prioritize mindfulness, nutrition, and movement can lead to a more energized, focused, and fulfilling life.

A morning routine is not just about waking up; it's about how we wake up. By practicing mindfulness the moment we open our eyes, we shift from a reactive to a proactive state. Techniques like deep breathing and visualization help center our thoughts, reduce stress, and cultivate a sense of purpose. The simple act of starting the day with controlled breathing can significantly impact our mental clarity and emotional stability. Rather than allowing external stimuli—emails, messages, or news alerts—to dictate our first thoughts, we can take charge of our mindset by setting positive intentions.

Gratitude and affirmations reinforce this mental shift. Expressing gratitude, whether through journaling or quiet reflection, nurtures a sense of contentment and appreciation, which in turn fosters resilience. When we start the day acknowledging what we are grateful for, we create a perspective that is rooted in positivity rather than stress or dissatisfaction. Similarly, daily affirmations act as gentle reminders of our capabilities, instilling confidence and motivation. By affirming our strengths and potential, we reprogram our minds to approach challenges with optimism rather than self-doubt.

Physical movement, no matter how minimal, is another crucial aspect of a balanced morning. Stretching, yoga, or light exercise awaken the body, improve circulation, and release endorphins— our natural mood boosters. The benefits of movement extend beyond just feeling awake; they contribute to long-term flexibility, muscle health, and overall vitality. The beauty of incorporating stretches or simple workouts into our morning routine is that it requires little time yet yields lasting benefits. Movement also encourages a smoother transition from sleep inertia to full alertness, ensuring that we step into the day with renewed energy rather than sluggishness.

Of course, what we put into our bodies in the morning plays a pivotal role in sustaining this energy. The importance of healthy fats as the first meal of the day cannot be overstated. Contrary to outdated beliefs that fats should be avoided, they are actually an essential source of sustainable energy. Ghee, for instance, provides nourishment while supporting digestion, enhancing metabolism, and promoting hormonal balance. Other alternatives like coconut oil, olive oil, and avocado offer similar benefits, ensuring that the body receives high-quality fuel rather than quick-burning carbohydrates that lead to energy crashes. A breakfast rich in healthy fats helps stabilize blood sugar levels, curbing mid-morning cravings and keeping the mind sharp.

Another powerful addition to a morning wellness regimen is the turmeric-ginger tea or shot. This golden elixir, packed with anti-inflammatory and immune-boosting properties, is an excellent way to support overall health. Turmeric and ginger work in harmony to reduce inflammation, aid digestion, and improve circulation, making them ideal choices for starting the day on a nourishing note. Their combined benefits create a protective shield against illnesses while enhancing gut health, which is integral to overall well-being.

These mindful morning habits — breathing, affirmations, movement, and nutrition — aren't just individual acts; they form a holistic system that lays the foundation for a healthier, happier life. When we prioritize our well-being first thing in the morning, we cultivate resilience, focus, and emotional balance. Instead of operating on autopilot, reacting to daily stressors, or feeling perpetually drained, we gain control over our time and energy.

Moreover, the beauty of a morning routine is its flexibility. While some people may thrive with meditation and elaborate journaling, others may find their rhythm in a simple cup of tea and a few moments of quiet reflection. The key is not perfection but consistency. Even small changes, like avoiding screens upon waking or drinking a warm glass of water before coffee, can have a profound impact over time.

At its core, a well-structured morning routine is an act of self-respect. It is a declaration that our well-being matters, that we deserve to begin our days with intention rather than chaos. When we take the time to nourish our bodies, center our minds, and move with purpose, we empower ourselves to handle life's challenges with greater ease. Our mornings are no longer an afterthought; they become a sacred space where we cultivate the energy and mindset necessary to thrive.

So, as you move forward, consider how you can tailor your mornings to support your goals and well-being. Whether you start by incorporating deep breathing, swapping out sugary breakfasts for healthy fats, or embracing the healing power of turmeric-ginger tea, know that every small step contributes to a larger transformation. The journey toward a healthier, more fulfilling life begins with a single morning—and the choice to make it intentional. You deserve mornings that energize and uplift you. You deserve a day that starts on your terms.

The Midday Meal—Finding Balance in Lunch

Lunch—oh, the meal that falls right in the middle of our hectic days, yet often gets overlooked or sabotaged by that 3:00 pm slump. It's the underdog of meals, sandwiched between the hectic hustle of breakfast and the comfort of dinner, yet it's arguably the most important meal of the day. But before we dive into the whirlwind world of meal prep, balanced bowls, and mindful indulgence, let's establish one undeniable fact: lunch deserves the spotlight.

Think about it. You wake up (begrudgingly, we know) to breakfast, a quick fix to jump-start your day, but by lunchtime, you're already running on fumes. The caffeine has worn off, and the morning's to-do list is still haunting you. This is where lunch comes in, offering the promise of energy and productivity... *if* you approach it correctly. If you skip lunch or worse, overwhelm your body with too much food, get ready for a ride of sluggishness, irritability, and bloated regrets. Trust me, we've all been there.

Skipping lunch is like trying to drive a car with an empty tank—eventually, you're going to stall. Your energy plummets, your mind starts wandering, and that afternoon dip turns into a free-fall. Productivity becomes a joke, and focus? Say goodbye to that. On the flip side, overloading at lunch is no better. Sure, the food might taste amazing, but your body's not exactly thrilled about the five-course meal you just forced it to process while it's trying to get back to work. Next thing you know, you're fighting a food coma and your only productivity is trying to keep your eyelids from doing their best impression of a blackout.

So why is lunch *that* important? It's simple. Lunch is the anchor that stabilizes your energy levels for the rest of the day. It ensures you're not hitting the dreaded 3:00 pm wall with an empty stomach and a frustrated mind. If you make the right choices, you'll stay energized, sharp, and more focused. It's like giving your brain and body the fuel it deserves to get through the rest of the day. Plus, let's be real—eating lunch is the perfect excuse to take a break from your never-ending to-do list and refresh your brain for a bit. If nothing else, lunch provides that much-needed mental reset.

In this chapter, we'll explore three main themes that will completely change your lunch game. First, we'll dive into meal gaps, why not taking proper breaks between meals leaves you feeling worse, and how you can keep your energy steady throughout the day. Then, we'll look at balanced meals and why it's not just about filling your plate with whatever's left in the fridge, but about giving your body the right nutrients to thrive. Lastly, we'll talk about mindful indulgence, because let's face it—nobody wants to feel guilty for enjoying a delicious treat at lunch. Moderation is key, and learning how to indulge without overdoing it can be a game-changer for both your health and happiness.

So buckle up, because your lunch routine is about to get a makeover that will keep you thriving, not just surviving.

The Science of Meal Gaps and Fasting

We've all been there—scrolling through Instagram while gnawing on a granola bar or grabbing a quick bite of something to quell that gnawing feeling in our stomachs between meals. But here's the thing: those little snack attacks? They might just be sabotaging your energy and digestion. It turns out that meal gaps—the time between breakfast, lunch, and dinner—are a big deal when it comes to feeling good and staying healthy. Your body, believe it or not, needs these breaks to recharge and, more importantly, to process the food you've already eaten.

First, let's talk about fat utilization. When you give your body the proper time between meals, it doesn't just sit there idly; it's burning fat to fuel your day. Yes, you read that right! You're essentially giving your metabolism a green light to tap into those fat stores for energy. Without enough time between meals, your body doesn't have the chance to burn through stored fat and ends up relying on what's in your bloodstream — i.e., sugars and carbs. So, next time you're thinking of munching away before your stomach even has time to fully process your last meal, consider that you might be robbing your body of the chance to burn fat.

And then there's the digestive system. Just like how we all need a break after a long day of work, your stomach, too, needs some downtime. Constantly feeding it can overwhelm your digestive tract, leaving you bloated, sluggish, and uncomfortable. Think of your stomach as a hardworking employee that deserves a little rest. You wouldn't want to keep your assistant on overtime 24/7, would you? Give your digestive system a break by spacing out meals with proper gaps. Your body will thank you by digesting more efficiently and making you feel lighter and more energized.

Now, the ideal gap is usually around 4-6 hours between meals. This window gives your body enough time to burn off the food you've already consumed, while preventing hunger pangs from spiraling out of control. But what happens if the gap is too short or too long? Well, if you're eating too frequently, your body doesn't have enough time to tap into its fat reserves, and you end up in a constant cycle of glucose-burning. On the flip side, if there's too much time between meals, you might find yourself turning into a ravenous beast when the next meal rolls around — hello, overeating and bloating.

How Fasting or Meal Gaps Affect the Body

Let's dive into the science behind those precious gaps. When we talk about meal gaps or fasting, we're really talking about regulating insulin and blood sugar levels. Insulin is the hormone that helps process sugar and fat in your body. If you're eating constantly, your body is in a state of high insulin, and that can lead to fat storage instead of fat burning. But when you maintain healthy meal gaps, you give your body time to reset, so it doesn't stay in a constant "fat-storing" mode. Your insulin levels drop, and this allows your body to switch to burning fat for energy, which is exactly what you want.

But that's not all. Proper meal timing also helps regulate blood sugar. If you eat too frequently or binge on sugary snacks, your blood sugar spikes, which is a one-way ticket to feeling sluggish and irritable. By maintaining a reasonable gap between meals, you avoid those sudden blood sugar crashes that make you reach for the nearest candy bar. The right amount of time between meals also helps keep your energy levels more stable throughout the day.

Meal gaps can also play a significant role in preventing overeating. When you eat too often, your body doesn't have the chance to properly register hunger cues. But when you space meals apart, your body gets time to digest, allowing your brain to properly signal when you're truly hungry. So, by the time the next meal rolls around, you're eating because your body *needs* food, not because your mind just can't handle the boredom.

The key to keeping your metabolism running like a well-oiled machine is timing. Skipping meals or eating too often can mess with your metabolism. But sticking to a healthy meal gap routine boosts metabolism by ensuring that your body can digest properly and utilize fat stores for energy instead of constantly working overtime to process the next round of food. This keeps your metabolism high and steady, meaning more energy and less effort for your body.

Practical Tips for Maintaining Healthy Gaps

So, now that we know meal gaps are essential, how do we maintain them? Don't worry, we've got you covered with some practical tips that are easy to implement (and maybe even a little fun).

First, let's talk about the snack trap. It's so easy to reach for that bag of chips or a sugary snack between meals, but those little indulgences throw off your timing. The key here is to avoid snacks that derail your meal gaps, particularly those sugary treats and refined carbs that give you a temporary sugar high followed by a crash. If you're feeling like you might just die of hunger between lunch and dinner, it's better to have a snack that won't ruin your metabolic rhythm. Opt for healthier, more substantial options — think nuts, seeds, or fruits. These are great choices because they're packed with healthy fats and fiber, giving your body a little something to work with without wreaking havoc on your blood sugar levels.

If you're finding it tricky to stave off cravings, consider water or herbal teas as your secret weapon. Hydration is key to managing hunger between meals. Sometimes, thirst can masquerade as hunger, so sipping on water or a calming tea can help curb those cravings and keep you hydrated. Herbal teas like chamomile or peppermint can also work wonders in relaxing your digestive system between meals, helping to keep everything running smoothly.

Now, what happens if you do need to snack? Don't panic! It's not about depriving yourself, but rather about being mindful of what you eat. Stick to nutrient-dense snacks that keep you full and satisfied without throwing off your metabolism. A handful of almonds, some fresh berries, or a few slices of apple with almond butter can tide you over without sending your blood sugar on a roller coaster ride. These snacks provide a balanced combination of healthy fats, protein, and fiber, all of which will keep you feeling full and energized, not sluggish and bloated.

Lastly, remember that the goal is mindful eating. Don't eat just because it's "time" or out of habit. Tune into your body's signals and listen to when you're genuinely hungry. Eating with intention and purpose will not only help you maintain proper meal gaps but will also make your meals more satisfying. Plus, there's something deeply satisfying about sitting down for a proper meal after giving your body the time to really process the last one.

So, there you have it! Maintaining healthy meal gaps is crucial for your energy, digestion, and metabolism. Give your body the breaks it deserves, resist the snack attack, and nourish it with the right food when hunger strikes. Your digestive system—and your mood—will thank you for it!

The Power of a Balanced Lunch

Ah, lunch—the glorious midday feast that has the power to either make or break your afternoon. It's the meal that can either fuel your productivity or leave you drooling over your keyboard in a food coma. So, how do we ensure that our lunch sets us up for success? Simple: by making it balanced. Think of a balanced lunch as your superhero cape, ready to fight off hunger, fatigue, and that overwhelming urge to take a nap at 2 pm. In this section, we'll explore the essential elements of a balanced lunch, from the sustaining carbs that power your day to the veggies that keep things running smoothly. Let's get into it!

High-Carb but Balanced: Grains as the Midday Star

Okay, I know what you're thinking—carbs, the villain of many a diet. But wait, before you throw your hands up in despair and declare a carb-free lunch, hear me out. Grains are not the enemy; in fact, they're your best friend, especially when it comes to lunch. Grains provide sustained energy and satiety, meaning you'll feel full and energized long after that final bite. Think of them as your lunch's reliable sidekick. They step in, do their job, and keep you feeling great until dinner.

But let's get specific. Whole grains—like whole wheat, brown rice, quinoa, and millet—are the champions here. Why? Because they're packed with fiber, which helps slow the digestion of sugars, keeping your blood sugar stable and preventing those dreaded afternoon crashes. Plus, they keep you full, so you're not eyeing the snack drawer two hours after lunch.

Now, portion control is important, and here's the rule of thumb: about 30-40% of your plate should be grains. This doesn't mean your plate should look like an all-you-can-eat buffet of rice or quinoa—balance is key. A modest serving is all you need to keep your energy levels soaring without tipping into carb overload. So, when you load up on your grain of choice, just remember: moderation, my friend.

The Vegetable Equation: Fiber, Vitamins, and Color

Here's where the magic happens. You've got your grains to fuel you, but vegetables are the secret sauce that takes your lunch from "meh" to "wow." Let's face it—if you're not eating enough veggies, you're doing yourself a disservice. Vegetables are the nutrient-dense powerhouses that deliver vitamins, minerals, fiber, and antioxidants—all the good stuff that keeps your body in tip-top shape. And the best part? They're naturally low in calories, which means you can pile them on your plate without guilt. If grains are your lunch's sidekick, veggies are your superhero team.

Here's the general rule: half your plate should be filled with vegetables. Yes, half. And no, you don't need to turn your lunch into a salad bar, but a variety of colorful veggies should make up the majority of your plate. Leafy greens, like spinach and kale, are packed with iron and calcium, while cruciferous vegetables like broccoli and cauliflower are known for their cancer-fighting properties. And don't forget about root vegetables, like carrots and sweet potatoes, which are full of vitamins and fiber.

Now, you might be wondering about cooking methods. Do you steam them? Roast them? Stir-fry them with a little bit of oil and seasoning? Yes to all of the above, depending on your preference. Light steaming, roasting, and stir-frying are all excellent ways to cook vegetables while preserving their nutrients. Roasting can bring out the natural sweetness of root vegetables, and stir-frying can add some tasty crunch without losing the vitamins. So, go ahead, experiment with cooking methods, and give your veggies the attention they deserve!

Protein as the Lunch Hero

Now, let's talk about the true hero of lunch: protein. Protein is crucial for tissue repair, muscle growth, and, of course, that wonderful feeling of fullness that keeps you from reaching for snacks. Without enough protein, you'll be left feeling hangry and unsatisfied, and trust me, nobody wants that.

For non-vegetarians, options like chicken, fish, and eggs are excellent sources of lean protein. These options are not only filling but also packed with essential amino acids that your body craves. Chicken breast, for example, is a low-fat, high-protein powerhouse that will keep you feeling full without the guilt.

For vegetarians, don't worry! You've got plenty of options, too. Lentils, beans, paneer, and tofu are all fantastic sources of plant-based protein. They're high in fiber, making them filling and great for digestion. Plus, they're super versatile—you can toss them in a curry, stir-fry them, or make a hearty lentil soup. The beauty of plant-based protein is that it's not just about getting full; it's about getting full while still fueling your body with fiber, vitamins, and minerals.

When it comes to portions, aim for about 20-25% of your plate to be dedicated to protein. This ensures you get enough to keep your muscles happy and your hunger at bay without overloading your digestive system.

Roti, Rice, or Both: Balancing Grains and Sides

Here's the age-old question: Roti or rice? For many of us, it's a decision we face every day, and depending on your mood, your hunger levels, or cultural preferences, you might gravitate toward one or the other. So, what's the right choice? Well, that depends on a few factors—your dietary preferences, your activity levels, and, of course, portion control.

Roti, made from whole wheat flour, is a great option if you're looking for a fiber boost and a lighter carb choice. It's perfect for those who want to avoid the heavy feeling that can come from eating too much rice. On the other hand, rice—especially brown rice or wild rice—gives you that satisfying, fluffy base for your meal, and it's a great choice if you're about to embark on a physically demanding afternoon. The key is balance. There's no need to have both roti and rice at the same meal unless you're really, really hungry or preparing for a marathon.

Cultural and regional preferences play a significant role here too. In some parts of the world, a lunch without rice is like a day without sunshine. But don't get too carried away; while rice is delicious and comforting, it's easy to overdo it. You want to be careful with portions to avoid a carb overload. Remember, moderation is your friend.

Putting It All Together

A balanced lunch isn't just about throwing random ingredients on a plate and calling it a day. It's about thoughtfully combining grains, vegetables, and protein in a way that supports your energy levels, digestion, and overall well-being. Fill half your plate with nutrient-packed veggies, about a third with hearty whole grains, and a quarter with protein—whether it's animal-based or plant-based. And don't forget to balance your carbs wisely with roti or rice—just remember to keep the portions in check.

By giving each food group its due time to shine, you'll create a lunch that not only keeps you full but also fuels your afternoon productivity without the post-lunch slump. So, next time you're planning your midday meal, remember: balance is the key to lunch success. Your body—and your productivity—will thank you!

The 80/20 Rule — Balance, Not Perfection

Let's face it: we all have that one food (or maybe a few) that we just can't quit. For some, it's pizza. For others, it's chocolate. And for some brave souls, it's even... French fries. The point is, while we strive for healthy eating habits, there's no reason to completely ditch those indulgent pleasures that make life *delicious*. Enter: the 80/20 rule. This magical principle doesn't just apply to investing or your work-life balance—it's the key to a balanced life in the kitchen as well. Let's break it down and figure out how to balance a wholesome lunch with the occasional treat, without feeling like you're sacrificing the good stuff. Spoiler alert: it's all about moderation and knowing when to splurge.

What is the 80/20 Rule?

Alright, here's the deal. The 80/20 rule is simple: 80% of your food intake should be wholesome, nutritious, and good-for-you foods, while the other 20% can be indulgent treats. That means you get to fill most of your plate with nutrient-packed grains, veggies, and proteins that nourish your body, and the remaining 20% is your *golden ticket* to enjoying your favorite less-than-healthy foods—without guilt.

Now, before you start imagining a life of perpetual restriction, let's clarify. The 80/20 rule isn't about depriving yourself; it's about balance and sustainability. You know, the kind of balance where you can eat your salad, feel great, and then enjoy that chocolate cake for dessert without immediately feeling like you've undone all your hard work. Because, let's be honest—life's too short to not have dessert every now and then. The trick is to embrace the 80% wholesome meals and allow yourself the 20% indulgence, without stressing over it.

Why does this approach work? Because it's sustainable! You're not setting yourself up for failure by going on extreme diets or making food feel like an enemy. Instead, you're creating a long-term habit of mindful eating, which means you're more likely to stick to it and feel happy with your choices. It's about knowing that today's healthy lunch can coexist with tomorrow's pizza night. Balance, my friends, balance.

Healthy Meals, with Room for Treats

Imagine this: You're sitting down to lunch. You've made yourself a well-rounded meal full of whole grains, veggies, and a good dose of protein. You're feeling pretty proud of yourself. But then, it hits you—you're craving a little something extra. Maybe it's a slice of pizza or a bowl of pasta with *extra cheese*. Don't panic! The beauty of the 80/20 rule is that your balanced lunch doesn't mean waving goodbye to your favorite foods forever.

Let's talk about incorporating healthier versions of classic "unhealthy" options. It's all about the swaps! You can still have the things you love, but you don't have to be reckless about it. For example:

- Adding veggies to your pasta or noodles: Ever thought about tossing a few spinach leaves or zucchini ribbons into your pasta? Suddenly, you've got some fiber, vitamins, and a burst of color on your plate. It's a small tweak, but it makes your meal feel like a healthier choice—without skimping on the flavor.

- Swapping regular burgers with whole-grain buns and grilled patties: Burgers, anyone? Sure, you could go for the classic fast-food version, but what if you swapped that soft, white bread bun for a hearty whole-grain one? And that deep-fried patty? Try grilling it instead. Your burger just got an upgrade — same juicy flavor, just a little more goodness going on. You might even *feel superior* as you munch away.

It's all about finding those little hacks that allow you to indulge without throwing your nutrition completely out the window. You don't have to give up your favorite foods; you just have to think smarter. Whether it's baking instead of frying, using whole grains instead of refined ones, or adding extra veggies to bulk up your meal, these changes don't make you a health freak — they just make you a smart foodie. And who doesn't want to be a smart foodie?

Fast Food and Treats: A Treat, Not a Habit

Ah, fast food. The love of our lives when we're in a hurry, the comfort we crave on a lazy Friday night. But before you start feeling guilty for enjoying a burger or a slice of pizza, remember this: treats are meant to be enjoyed, not feared. The problem arises when we make fast food or unhealthy snacks a regular habit instead of an occasional treat. It's the difference between treating yourself after a stressful week and scarfing down fast food every day because you're "too tired to cook."

The beauty of the 80/20 rule is that it allows you to indulge, but in a way that doesn't derail your goals. So, next time you're craving those crispy fries or that cheesy pizza, remember: you're not breaking any rules. You're simply partaking in mindful indulgence.

Here's the key: enjoying fast food without guilt. Yes, you can savor that pizza without feeling like your entire week of healthy eating has been erased. In fact, occasional indulgences can have positive effects on both your physical and mental well-being. That burger?

It's not just food — it's a little moment of joy, a reminder that life is about enjoying the *whole experience* (including food) in moderation. So go ahead, enjoy that treat — just don't make it your daily habit.

Now, how do you indulge without going overboard? Here are a few tips for smarter indulgences:

1. Choose smaller portions: You don't need the large fries or the jumbo-sized burger. Opt for a smaller portion and still get that satisfying flavor without the overload. After all, size matters — just not in the way you think!
2. Share your treat: If you're dining with friends or family, why not share? That way, you get a taste of your favorite food, but you're not indulging in the entire thing. Plus, it's more fun to share food with others (and you get to say things like, "Don't worry, I'll take the last bite").
3. Pair with healthier sides: If you're grabbing fast food, balance things out with a healthier option on the side. Maybe a side salad, or a fresh juice instead of a sugary soda. You're still getting your treat, but you're also sneaking in a little extra nutrition.

At the end of the day, the 80/20 rule is about freedom — freedom to enjoy your favorite foods without guilt, freedom to eat nutritious meals that fuel your body, and freedom to live without food dictating your life. It's about balance and enjoying life in all its deliciousness, without stressing over every bite. So, the next time you reach for that piece of cake or a side of fries, know that it's just part of your 20%. You've got your 80% covered — and that's what truly matters.

Remember, life's too short to live in a food prison. Embrace balance, enjoy the treats, and trust that your body will thank you for it. Now, go ahead and have that chocolate. You've earned it!

Structuring a Balanced Plate (Visual and Practical Guide)

We've all seen those perfectly styled food photos on Instagram, with vibrant greens, rich grains, and a delicious-looking protein — all stacked artfully on a plate that somehow seems to make even our own kitchen creations look like amateur hour. But the truth is, building a balanced plate doesn't need to be a food stylist's dream come true — it can be a simple, everyday process that gives you the energy and satisfaction to take on the rest of your day. Whether you're a seasoned meal prep pro or just someone trying to survive lunchtime without a frantic scramble, let's break down the essentials of crafting a balanced plate that's easy on the eyes and even easier on your stomach.

Building Your Perfect Plate: Approximate Percentages

Now, we're not talking about some complex equation or a Pinterest-perfect masterpiece — this is real food for real people, and it's all about getting the right components on your plate in the right amounts. So, let's take a closer look at the ideal ratios:

- Grains (30-40%): Grains are the foundation of your plate — they're like the solid backbone of a good story. Think rice, quinoa, brown rice, or even couscous. These provide the energy you need to power through your afternoon and keep your stomach from grumbling like a bear on a fast. Now, don't go overboard here — 30-40% is the sweet spot. More than that, and you're looking at a plate full of carbs, with less room for all the other delicious and nutritious components.

- Vegetables (50%): Half of your plate should be filled with vegetables. Not only do they make your plate look like a rainbow, but they're also packed with fiber, vitamins, and minerals that help keep your digestive system running smoothly. And don't be afraid to mix it up—leafy greens, cruciferous vegetables (hello, broccoli!), root vegetables, and everything in between. Plus, you'll be left feeling full, but not weighed down—like you've just eaten a salad but also a satisfying, hearty meal. Try adding a mix of raw and cooked vegetables to keep things interesting (and maybe throw in a little roasted sweet potato for some extra flair).

- Protein (20-25%): Protein is your power player in this game. It helps with muscle repair, keeps you full, and basically helps prevent you from turning into a hangry mess around 3 pm. Whether you're a carnivore or a plant lover, there's a protein source for everyone. Think chicken, fish, eggs, tofu, lentils, beans, or paneer. Don't overload here either—keep it around 20-25% of your plate so that you're not eating a chicken leg *and* a side of fish *and* a tofu salad. One solid protein source is all you need.

- Fats (5-10%): Ah, fats. They make everything taste better, don't they? A little goes a long way when it comes to healthy fats—think ghee, olive oil, nuts, or seeds. A small drizzle of olive oil on your veggies or a spoonful of ghee on your rice can take your meal from "meh" to "mmm." Not to mention, fats help with the absorption of fat-soluble vitamins like A, D, E, and K, so don't skimp on them. But don't go pouring a vat of oil—keep it around 5-10% of your plate.

Regional Examples of Balanced Plates

Now that we've talked about the components of a balanced plate, let's take a quick tour around the world and look at some regional examples. You'll see that balance isn't just a western concept—it's something that's embedded in cuisines all over the globe. Here are a few examples to get you thinking:

- Indian Thali: The Indian thali is the gold standard of a balanced plate. You've got dal (lentils) for protein, roti (whole wheat flatbread) or rice for your grains, sabzi (vegetable curry) for those vital veggies, and raita (yogurt with cucumber and spices) for a refreshing, cool touch. It's a meal that checks all the boxes for nutrition, flavor, and satisfaction. Just be careful with that extra helping of dal — while it's delicious, too much might make you feel like you need a nap.

- Mediterranean Plate: If you're ever unsure what to eat for lunch, the Mediterranean plate is a safe bet. Grilled fish (hello, omega-3s) pairs beautifully with quinoa, fresh salad, and a scoop of hummus. The Mediterranean diet has long been praised for its heart-healthy benefits, and it's easy to see why — it's full of fresh ingredients, healthy fats, and lean proteins. Plus, it's all about enjoying your food slowly, so go ahead, take your time with that hummus.

- Asian-Inspired Bowl: Picture this: a steaming bowl of brown rice (hello, fiber), topped with stir-fried veggies (everything from bell peppers to bok choy) and your choice of tofu or chicken. A drizzle of sesame dressing ties it all together. This Asian-inspired bowl is a perfect balance of grains, veggies, and protein, with the added bonus of some healthy fats from the sesame oil. It's fresh, light, and comforting all at once.

Prepping Ahead for Lunchtime Success

We've all been there: it's noon, and you're staring into your fridge, hoping some food will magically appear. But instead, you're left wondering if you should just order delivery or eat yet another sad sandwich. Trust me, we've all been in that "what's for lunch?" panic mode. The solution? Meal prep. It's your new best friend.

The key to a successful lunch is not just having the right ingredients — it's also about having them ready when hunger strikes. Here are a few meal prep strategies to save you from lunchtime chaos:

1. Plan and Prep: Start by creating a meal plan for the week. Take time to organize your grocery list, ensuring you have all the ingredients you need for balanced, nutritious meals. Dedicate one day (like Sunday) to meal prep—wash, chop, and portion your veggies, cook a batch of grains, and prep proteins. Having everything ready to go makes assembling meals quick and stress-free, helping you stay on track with healthy eating.
2. Simple Recipes for Variety: You don't need to reinvent the wheel each day. Cook a large batch of something like roasted sweet potatoes, grilled chicken, or chickpeas, and then mix and match with different veggies, sauces, and grains. Throw in some avocado or a handful of nuts for extra flavor and texture. That way, even though you're eating similar ingredients, your lunch will feel fresh every day.
3. Get Creative with Leftovers: Leftovers are your best friend in the world of meal prep. Take that extra chicken from last night's dinner and turn it into a wrap or salad for lunch. Or if you've got leftover veggies, toss them into a frittata or mix them with quinoa for a quick bowl. The beauty of leftovers is that they save time and reduce food waste—so don't throw away that extra rice or those last bits of roasted veggies. They're gold for your next meal.

Lunch Beyond the Plate—Mindful Eating Habits

You've got your perfectly balanced lunch, your grains, your greens, and your protein, but wait—there's one last piece of the puzzle: mindful eating. It's not just about what's on your plate; it's about how you approach it. Let's dive into some mindful eating habits that could transform your lunch break into something much more than just a mid-day refueling.

The Importance of Eating Slowly

Ever eaten lunch so quickly that by the time you're done, you're already planning your next meal and wondering where it all went? Yep, guilty as charged. Here's the thing: eating slowly isn't just for people who are fancy or Zen masters; it's actually a game-changer for your digestion and overall well-being.

First off, eating slowly gives your digestive system a chance to actually digest. It's not a race. You don't need to inhale your food like you're preparing for a competitive eating contest. When you slow down, your body has time to produce the digestive enzymes and stomach acids it needs to break down your food properly. It also helps prevent overeating. Ever gone to a buffet and piled your plate high, only to realize halfway through that you're stuffed? That's because your brain and gut are in a race to communicate. By eating slowly, you're giving your brain enough time to catch up and send the "Hey, we're full" signal before you've consumed half your body weight in lasagna.

Now, why does it take 20 minutes to feel full? Welcome to the brain-gut connection. Your gut is a bit like the late-night party guest who shows up, has a blast, but takes their sweet time to let the host (your brain) know they're ready to go home. When you eat slowly, your stomach stretches, and it sends signals to your brain that it's had enough. If you eat too quickly, your brain hasn't had enough time to get the memo. So, next time you're scarfing down a sandwich in record time, remember: eating slowly means your stomach and brain are throwing a dinner party together—and you want them to enjoy it without any miscommunications.

Creating a Lunchtime Ritual

Let's face it, lunch isn't always the highlight of your day when you're eating at your desk, with your laptop open, trying to respond to emails while simultaneously managing to get some food in your mouth. But eating at your desk is like multitasking at its worst—it's stressful, it's unsatisfying, and your brain doesn't get a proper break. Your lunch break is the perfect opportunity to step away from the chaos of the day and create a little ritual.

So, step one: sit down. Yes, actually sit down at a table or a comfy spot and make it a moment of peace. Step two: disconnect from your screens. It's a simple, revolutionary act that will make you feel like you're living in the future. Trust me, your email can wait 20 minutes, and the social media updates will still be there after you finish your meal.

Now, here's where it gets really fun. Add a small ritual. Maybe you take a moment to give thanks for the meal before you dig in, or simply take a few deep breaths before you start eating. No, you don't need to be chanting "om" or practicing yoga poses while you chew (unless you want to, in which case, go ahead), but taking a moment to mindfully chew your food can make a big difference. Try to chew each bite slowly, savoring the flavors, and noticing the texture. By engaging your senses, you'll feel more satisfied with less food, and your body will thank you for it.

And if you want to take it a step further, you can use your lunchtime to catch up with a friend or coworker and enjoy your meal together. No rush, no stress—just a peaceful break from the hustle.

Mindful eating is all about being present in the moment with your food. Eating slowly helps you digest better, feel fuller with less food, and makes the whole experience more enjoyable. Creating a lunchtime ritual, on the other hand, is your secret weapon for turning a simple meal into a well-deserved break that recharges you for the rest of the day. So next time you sit down for lunch, remember to savor it, disconnect from the chaos, and maybe even say a little thank-you to that delicious sandwich for keeping you going.

The Science of Lunch and Overall Health

We've all been there: it's 3 PM, and suddenly you're struggling to keep your eyes open, your brain feels like it's wading through molasses, and your body is staging a quiet protest against productivity. What's going on? The culprit could be your lunch — or lack of a balanced one. Let's dive into how a well-structured lunch can save you from that dreaded afternoon slump and provide long-term health benefits.

Blood Sugar and Energy Regulation

Ah, the afternoon slump — that magical time of day when your energy levels plummet faster than your motivation to work. But here's the thing: a balanced lunch can actually be the hero of your midday malaise. The secret is in your blood sugar levels. When you chow down on a lunch full of simple carbs (we're talking that white bread sandwich or sugary pasta), you get a quick surge of energy. It's like a sugar high followed by a crashing low, making you feel sluggish and irritable. Not exactly the productivity boost you were hoping for.

Enter complex carbs and protein — the dynamic duo that keeps your blood sugar levels stable and your energy flowing evenly. When you eat whole grains, beans, and vegetables (those lovely complex carbs), your body breaks them down slowly, releasing a steady stream of energy. Meanwhile, protein (think chicken, beans, or tofu) helps keep you feeling fuller for longer, so you're not eyeing the vending machine by 2:30 PM. Together, they help maintain those sweet, stable blood sugar levels, and that means no energy roller coasters. You'll have the stamina to power through the afternoon and still have enough mental energy left to enjoy your post-workday Netflix binge.

Mood and Productivity Boost

Now, let's talk about mood and productivity — two things that can go from "I'm on top of the world!" to "Please just let me nap" in a matter of hours. What you eat for lunch can have a huge impact on how your brain performs later on. Nutrient-dense foods — those that are rich in vitamins, minerals, fiber, and healthy fats — are like brain fuel. Your brain needs proper nutrition to keep your cognitive function sharp and your mood in check.

Skipping lunch or filling up on junk food can lead to irritability, brain fog, and a general sense of *meh*. Ever noticed how a bag of chips doesn't exactly lead to a surge of creativity? Instead, you're left wondering why you thought it was a good idea to eat that entire bag. When you choose nutrient-packed foods (like veggies, whole grains, and lean proteins), you'll be doing your brain and mood a huge favor. No more cranky, foggy afternoons. Just clear, focused energy and a generally happier you.

Long-Term Benefits of Balanced Lunches

The benefits of a balanced lunch aren't just short-term — your future self will thank you too. Long-term health is built on the choices you make today, and having a well-rounded lunch every day plays a key role in reducing the risk of chronic conditions like diabetes, obesity, and heart disease.

When you nourish your body with the right mix of nutrients, you're supporting gut health (hello, happy microbiome!), boosting metabolism, and keeping your energy levels stable. This reduces your chances of developing metabolic diseases down the road and can even help keep you at a healthy weight. Plus, a balanced diet supports your body's natural defenses, so you're more likely to avoid catching every cold that goes around.

Conclusion: Lunch as a Lifestyle

Alright, folks, let's wrap this up—because by now, your stomach is probably starting to remind you that it's time for a solid lunch. But before you grab whatever's closest, let's quickly revisit why lunch is so much more than just a pit stop between breakfast and dinner.

First, we talked about meal gaps. The key takeaway? Don't just eat on autopilot—give your body the space it needs between meals to function properly. It's not about starving yourself, but rather about making sure you're giving your digestive system the time it deserves to rest and reset. Plus, those 4-6 hours between meals? They give your body the chance to burn fat, regulate blood sugar, and, let's be honest, give you the energy to conquer the next task without feeling like you're going to pass out by 3 PM.

Then there's the balanced nutrition—we've covered the whole "grains, vegetables, protein" thing, and you've probably already heard this before, but here's the thing: it works. A solid lunch with a balanced plate is like your body's personal power-up. You're fueling not just your stomach, but also your brain. With the right mix of carbs, protein, and fats, you're setting yourself up for stable energy, improved mood, and the ability to actually focus on whatever you're doing. Gone are the days of crashing after lunch like a phone with 1% battery. It's all about that steady, long-lasting charge.

And let's not forget about indulgence. Yes, you read that right—indulgence. While we're all about balanced meals, it's also okay to take a little detour every now and then and enjoy something that brings you joy. Maybe it's a slice of cake, a crispy fry, or a cheesy quesadilla. The key here is moderation. Don't let food guilt sneak up on you like an uninvited guest at a dinner party. Instead, think of your occasional treat as a celebration of life and good taste. After all, food is meant to bring joy, not just serve as fuel.

So, what's the bottom line here? Lunch isn't just a meal — it's a lifestyle. It's the chance to pause, breathe, and give your body what it needs to keep you going through the day. It's your midday opportunity to nourish, energize, and even indulge (without guilt). View lunch as your personal opportunity to not just fuel your body, but to celebrate the simple joys of life. It's about making every bite count, whether it's a health-packed salad or a bowl of comfort food.

Remember: food is not just fuel — it's also a celebration. So, the next time you sit down for lunch, make it count. Mix in some health, sprinkle in a little taste, and top it off with a dash of happiness. That's how you create the perfect recipe for a balanced and fulfilling lunch — and maybe even a better day. Bon appétit!

The Snack Debate - When, What, and How Much?

In today's world, snacking has become less of a necessity and more of a full-on ritual. You walk into a store, and it's like a snack wonderland—chips, cookies, bars, and things you didn't even know could be snacks (gummy bears as a protein source, anyone?). It's safe to say snacking has taken over our lives. But here's the million-dollar question: Are we actually *hungry*, or are we just eating because it's the thing to do?

The rise of snacking is a symptom of our busy, always-on-the-go culture. We're juggling work, life, and 18 open tabs on our computers, and suddenly—boom—we're craving something to munch on, preferably something we can eat while scrolling through social media. It's easy to reach for a quick snack to fill the gap between meals, but let's be real—most of the time, we're not even hungry. We're just trying to escape that midday slump, avoid dealing with feelings of boredom, or distract ourselves from our endless to-do list.

Sure, snacks can be a life-saver when you're starving between meals, but often, they're just filling a void that has less to do with actual hunger and more to do with our need for instant gratification. Our bodies, when properly fueled at mealtime, are totally fine without that afternoon bag of chips. But somehow, we've convinced ourselves that if we don't snack, we're missing out on life's greatest pleasure—eating at *all* times of the day.

So, next time you reach for a snack, ask yourself: "Am I truly hungry, or am I just bored, stressed, or in need of a break?" Spoiler alert: If it's the latter, maybe it's time to rethink that bag of pretzels. Or, at least, pair it with something healthier.

Snacking and Lifestyle

The Active Lifestyle Snackers

If you're the kind of person who treats a 5K run like a warm-up or thinks a gym membership is an essential life investment, then you're probably well-acquainted with the magical power of snacks. For those who live an active lifestyle—whether you're pumping iron, running marathons, or climbing mountains (metaphorically or literally)—snacking isn't just a luxury; it's a necessity. Your body is basically a high-performance car, and like any high-end vehicle, it needs fuel to keep those engines revving.

Active individuals burn through energy quickly, and that's where snacks come in. After an intense workout, your body is craving protein to rebuild those muscles and carbs to refuel the energy stores you just emptied. Enter the magical snack: nuts, protein bars, smoothies, or even a good old-fashioned avocado toast (because, yes, we all know it's practically the official food of the active set). These snacks aren't just tasty—they're your workout's best friend. You need protein to help those muscles recover, healthy fats for sustained energy, and some carbs to keep your metabolism humming.

But, please, avoid the trap of reaching for that packet of chips just because it's sitting in front of you while you flex in the mirror. For active folks, snacks should be energy-boosting, not energy-sapping. Choose snacks that can actually help you level up your health game. So, think whole-grain energy bars, Greek yogurt with a handful of berries, or a smoothie packed with protein powder and healthy fats. Keep it smart, and your body will thank you by being able to take on whatever physical feat you throw at it—whether that's an intense HIIT session or running after the bus.

The Sedentary Lifestyle Snackers

Now, for the flip side — those of us who live life a little more... *relaxed*. You know the type: lounging on the couch after a long day, possibly engaged in an intense Netflix marathon or scrolling through endless TikTok videos. For these sedentary snackers, snacking takes on a different form, often one that's not so friendly to your waistline or digestion. The more you sit, the less energy your body burns, and yet, the snack attack still seems to hit at full force.

The problem with sedentary snacking is that it's easy to overeat, and the snacks we crave often aren't exactly nutrient-dense. Chips, cookies, and that half-finished chocolate bar you found buried in your purse — yep, those are the culprits. But here's the thing: if you're not burning off those calories, guess where they're going? That's right, straight to your waistline. And let's be honest, no one's going to be thrilled with their digestion after downing that entire bag of pretzels while watching a two-hour movie.

For the sedentary snackers, it's crucial to make better choices. Opt for snacks that are lighter, smaller in portion, and packed with nutrients — think fruits, Greek yogurt, or a handful of almonds. These will keep your body satisfied without the sugar crash and energy dip that follows eating processed snacks. You can also go for small servings of protein like a boiled egg or a few slices of turkey. These snacks help curb hunger and provide your body with what it needs without causing those unwanted afternoon energy crashes.

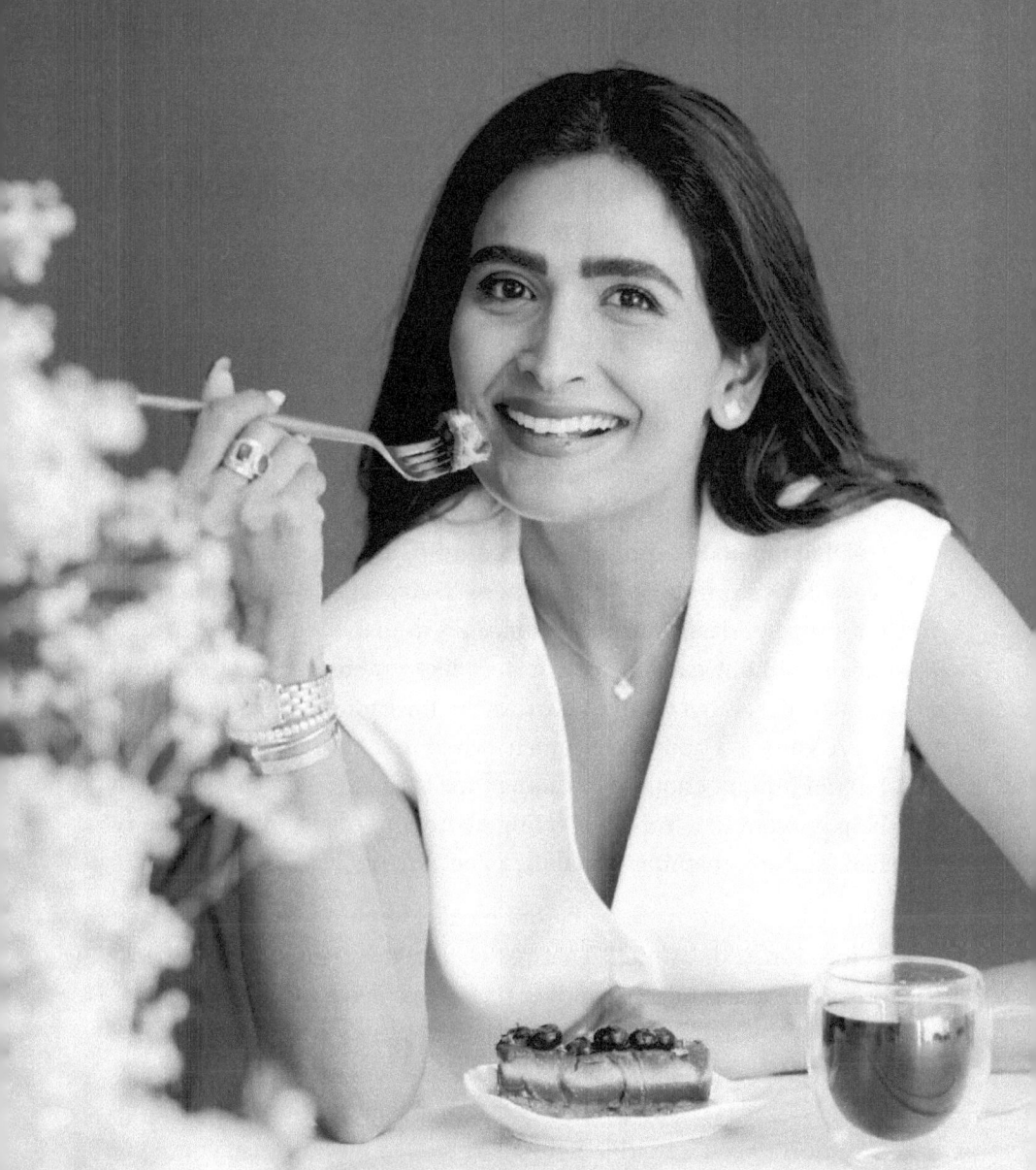

When to Snack?

Ah, timing — it's everything, right? Whether you're an active, health-conscious individual or someone who's just trying to survive the day without a meltdown, when you snack can make all the difference. The perfect snack timing is all about balancing your energy levels, your meal schedule, and, of course, your general life chaos.

Let's start with when to snack based on your meal timings. If you're having a nice, well-balanced breakfast and lunch, you're likely to feel that inevitable, mid-afternoon slump, the one where your brain feels like it's running on 10% battery. That's when you should reach for a snack. Ideally, a snack should fill in that energy gap between meals without causing you to feel like you're about to roll into dinner like an overstuffed burrito. So, the optimal time for a snack is typically 2-3 hours after lunch, when that "I'm not full anymore but not hungry enough for dinner" feeling hits. Snack time can also help prevent you from overeating at dinner because you've already had a little something to stabilize your energy levels.

But what about snacking before meals? Should you have a snack before lunch or dinner? That really depends. If you're not one to enjoy full meals and get hunger pangs that send you straight to the kitchen, a small snack before meals can curb your appetite. But don't go wild — save those snacks for when you're genuinely hungry, not as a way to avoid facing the fearsome task of cooking. You don't need a double helping of snacks just because you were "bored."

The Late-Night Snack Dilemma

Now, let's talk about the late-night snack dilemma. Everyone's been there: you're cozy on the couch, the day is winding down, and suddenly that irresistible urge to munch hits. Is it okay to have a snack right before bed? Well, sometimes. If you're staying up late and your stomach's doing backflips, then a light snack can settle your mind and your hunger. Go for something easy to digest: a handful of almonds, a small bowl of Greek yogurt with a drizzle of honey, or a piece of dark chocolate—something simple that won't leave you tossing and turning later.

On the other hand, if you're just snacking because you're mindlessly scrolling through your phone or trying to avoid feeling like a responsible adult, then just skip it. Late-night snacks that are heavy, greasy, or sugary can disrupt your sleep and mess with your metabolism. Plus, let's be real—no one ever wakes up from a midnight pizza binge feeling like they made good decisions.

Snack vs. Meal: How to Avoid Snacking Becoming a Meal

Ah, portion control. The eternal struggle. You tell yourself, "Just one handful of chips," and the next thing you know, you're standing over an empty bag, wondering how it all happened. Snack vs. meal is a very fine line to walk, and it's easy to cross it without realizing. Snacks are meant to be little pick-me-ups, not an entire meal replacement. While snacks should help keep your energy levels up, they're not meant to replace a proper meal, even if you're choosing the healthiest options.

So, how do you keep snacks in their rightful place? Portion control is key. Snack portions should be small, so they're more like a gentle pit stop rather than a detour that leads to the snack aisle of your local supermarket. If your snack feels like it could double as lunch, then you've probably crossed into meal territory. Stick to single servings, and if you find yourself still hungry after a snack, wait a bit before deciding to have another snack. Hydrate, too—sometimes your body just needs water, not more food.

Sweet vs. Savory: The Great Snack Debate

Sweet Snacks: The Tempting Sugar Rush

Let's be real, sweet snacks are the undisputed champions when it comes to satisfying those cravings. There's something almost magical about biting into a chocolate chip cookie or digging into a bowl of ice cream (let's face it, we've all been there). The appeal of sweet snacks lies in their ability to give you that instant rush of happiness, as if the world's problems could be solved by sugar alone. But before you dive headfirst into a sugar coma, let's think about it for a second.

Craving sugar isn't a crime—it's just biology. Your brain loves sugar because it provides that quick energy fix, but the problem is that the sweet stuff often gives you a sugar high followed by a crash that leaves you hunting for your next sugar fix like a zombie. This isn't the plot of a bad sitcom; it's your body trying to tell you something. Balance is key.

Some healthier, more affordable options to satisfy your sweet tooth without spiraling into a sugar abyss include things like fruit salads (hello, antioxidants!), dark chocolate (because you're fancy and health-conscious), or energy balls made with dried fruits and nuts (your own little snack-sized power pack). These alternatives don't spike your blood sugar as much, leaving you feeling full and satisfied without the regret that comes with a bag of gummy bears.

Remember, indulging in sweet snacks is fine—just be mindful of portions, and try to balance out those sugar spikes by pairing sweet snacks with fiber or healthy fats. If you're really feeling the craving, a few squares of dark chocolate (70% or higher, of course) can make your soul happy without overloading you with sugar.

Savory Snacks: The Unsung Heroes of Snacking

On the other side of the snack spectrum lies the humble savory snack. Often overshadowed by their sweet counterparts, savory snacks are the unsung heroes of the snacking world. These little morsels are often more satisfying and provide a longer-lasting energy boost than their sugar-filled siblings. Why? Because savory snacks tend to be a better balance of protein, fats, and carbs—the holy trinity that keeps your body satisfied and your stomach from growling at inappropriate times.

For savory snack lovers, think roasted chickpeas, hummus with veggie sticks, or crackers with cheese. These snacks are full of nutrients and will keep you going through that mid-afternoon slump without the crash that comes with sweets. Not only do they provide that satisfying "I'm full but not stuffed" feeling, but they're also great for your energy levels.

Healthy Indian and Western savory snacks include simple, affordable options like spiced roasted nuts, sundal (seasoned chickpeas), and samosa baked versions (because why fry when you can bake?). For the Western crowd, go for options like avocado toast or guacamole with whole-grain chips—because let's be honest, who doesn't love a good dip?

Savory snacks are particularly good for people who are more active or need a steady supply of energy throughout the day. Whether you're running errands, working, or even binge-watching your favorite show, a savory snack will keep your mind sharp and your energy steady.

Indian vs. Western Snacks

Indian Snack Culture: The Heart of Munching

Ah, Indian snacks—the glorious affair that begins in the late afternoon and sometimes doesn't end until you've had your third round of chai at 9 PM. Indian snacks are not just food; they're a lifestyle. Whether you're taking a break from work or casually bonding with friends, snacks are a key part of the day. They're the little bite-sized wonders that hold you over between meals—or in some cases, they become the meal.

The classic Indian snack experience involves a warm, satisfying treat like samosas, bhel puri, or chivda. Picture this: the spicy, tangy crunch of bhel puri or the crispiness of a perfectly fried samosa. It's heaven, right? But let's not forget that deep-frying comes with a price—high fat and oil content. Eating samosas might feel like you're devouring joy itself, but your waistline may not appreciate it as much. Roasted peanuts, a snack found in nearly every Indian home, are more than just a snack—they're a reminder that sometimes simplicity is perfection. Packed with protein, they can be your best friend during those 4 PM slumps. But beware! Eating them by the fistful might lead to more "slump" than you intended.

Making Indian Snacks Healthier

Now, I'm all for keeping tradition alive, but let's also be smart about it. You don't have to give up your beloved samosas and chivda, but you can make them healthier. Try baked samosas instead of deep-fried ones. You still get that satisfying crunch but with a fraction of the oil. Or, swap out some of the fried snacks for roasted chickpeas or veggie chivda—packed with protein and fiber, these alternatives will make you feel like you're eating something indulgent without the guilty aftermath.

For those who absolutely cannot imagine life without deep-fried snacks (we get you), at least try reducing the oil used. Just because it's deep-fried doesn't mean it should be floating in a pool of oil. And add more vegetables—your taste buds will be too busy savoring the flavors to even notice they're eating something *healthy*.

Western Snack Culture: Convenience Overload

Ah, the West. Where snacks are often smaller, but no less tempting. From chips to granola bars, these snacks are a masterclass in convenience. But here's the catch: many of them are a tad lacking in the nutritional department. Sure, a granola bar might sound healthy, but have you looked at the label? That seemingly innocent bar could be packed with enough added sugar to send you into a sugar coma before your next Zoom meeting.

But hey, let's not get too judgmental about Western snacks. We've all devoured a packet of chips when no one was looking. And while chips might be the snack equivalent of comfort food, they're not exactly a powerhouse of nutrients. For a more wholesome option, look for granola bars with minimal added sugar and ones that pack a punch with fiber, nuts, and seeds. Or, opt for veggie chips instead of your regular bag of fried potatoes — because sometimes, your body needs veggies, even if they come in the form of chips.

One of the biggest appeals of Western snacks is the pre-packaged convenience. While it's easy to grab a pack of cookies or a bag of chips, sometimes we have to remind ourselves that not all pre-packaged foods are bad. Look for healthier alternatives that are more about whole ingredients than preservatives and sugar. Nut butters, trail mixes, and whole-grain crackers with cheese are some examples of snacks that you can grab without regretting your life choices 20 minutes later.

Practical Tips for Smart Snacking

Planning Snacks Ahead: A Future You Will Thank

Let's be real: we've all been there. You're at work, and suddenly, it's snack o'clock. Your brain goes into autopilot mode, and before you know it, you've demolished an entire bag of chips while binge-watching cooking videos (we've all done it, don't pretend you haven't). This is where planning ahead can save you from yourself.

One of the easiest ways to avoid the impulse grab-and-go is to prepare and portion your snacks for the week. It sounds like a lot of work, but trust me, future you will appreciate not having to rush to the vending machine at 3 PM. Chop up some fruits, prep your homemade energy balls, or portion out servings of nuts into small containers. That way, when hunger strikes, you don't have to make decisions based on what's available—your snacks are already waiting for you.

Quick, easy, and affordable snack recipes could be something like overnight oats (mix oats, milk, and your favorite toppings, and boom, you've got a healthy snack for later) or chickpea salad (toss chickpeas with some olive oil, lemon, and your favorite spices). These snacks are simple, affordable, and keep you full, so you're not reaching for the cookie jar at the first sign of stress.

Mindful Snacking: The Art of Eating (Without the Guilt)

Let's get one thing straight: snacking isn't about mindlessly inhaling food. It's about enjoying the moment, the flavor, and the fact that you're nourishing your body (as opposed to just filling it with junk). Mindful snacking is exactly what it sounds like: eating with intention. Focus on the texture, taste, and aroma of your snack. If you're eating a handful of almonds, *feel* the crunch, *enjoy* the flavor, and savor the experience.

Mindfulness also means listening to your body's hunger cues. If you're snacking because you're bored, stressed, or avoiding work, maybe it's time to reassess. Sometimes the best snack is just water—your body might be thirsty, not hungry.

If you're reaching for a snack, ask yourself: Am I hungry? Or do I just need a distraction? Eating when you're genuinely hungry and not because you're bored or stressed will not only prevent overeating but will also make your snack feel more satisfying. And don't forget the portion control—no one needs a mountain of chips, no matter how good they smell.

Should You Skip Snacks?

Let's face it: snacking is a lifestyle. It's like that friend who always pops by uninvited, but you secretly love them because they make everything more fun. But sometimes, it's time to ask: *should we be snacking right now, or should we just let the chips (literally) fall where they may?*

There's definitely a time and place to skip the snack—and sometimes, the best snack is the one you don't eat. When your stomach is still full from a hearty meal, adding another snack just because it's "snack time" can lead to some serious bloating and a sluggish digestive system. It's like trying to jam one more episode into a Netflix binge when the show's already ended—no need to force it.

Another scenario where it's better to skip snacks? Mindless overeating. We've all been there, reaching for the snack bowl not because we're actually hungry, but because we're bored, stressed, or just plain *emotionally attached* to food. If you're in this habit, it's time to ask yourself: *Are you really hungry, or is your body just bored of Netflix too?* Constantly snacking without hunger can mess with your digestion and cause your body to go into "never-ending eating mode", making it hard to gauge when you're truly full.

Here's a simple test: Before you snack, pause and check in with your body. Ask yourself: *Is my stomach actually growling? Is there a physical need for energy, or am I just using food as a distraction?* If it's the latter, maybe take a 10-minute walk or drink a glass of water instead. You might find that your desire for a snack disappears once you've engaged in something that doesn't involve food.

Snacking with Purpose

Now that we've got the snacks sorted, let's get real about the ultimate takeaway: snack with purpose. Snacking doesn't need to be a mindless ritual—it can be an intentional, nourishing part of your day. When done thoughtfully, snacks can help you maintain energy, avoid hunger pangs, and even boost your mood. But—and this is a big but—you need to listen to your body. It's the most reliable snack advisor you'll ever have.

Balancing snacks with meals, timing them correctly, and choosing nutrient-dense options over junky fillers will set you up for success. Think of snacks as tools for your body: energy boosters, mood enhancers, and little moments of joy that can fuel your productivity and creativity. But just like any tool, they need to be used wisely. They shouldn't be a filler for something else—especially not boredom, stress, or the overpowering urge to procrastinate.

Remember, snacks are meant to nourish, not to become the center of your eating habits. A snack shouldn't be something you feel compelled to eat just because it's "snack time"—it should be something that makes you feel better, not worse. When you choose snacks based on your lifestyle, timing, and actual hunger, you'll find the right balance and make snacks a healthy, enjoyable, and effective part of your day.

So, the next time you're reaching for that snack, ask yourself: *Is this for real hunger or just for fun?* And if it's the former, enjoy it with intention—after all, snacking should be an experience, not a filler!

Dinner - The Final Meal of the Day

Ah, dinner—the grand finale of our daily food marathon. It's the last hurrah before we head into a night of relaxation, Netflix, or, if you're feeling fancy, pretending to read a book before passing out. But while dinner often feels like the "reward" after a long day, its significance goes beyond satisfying our taste buds and filling our stomachs. It's the meal that can determine how well we sleep, how we feel the next day, and even our overall health. Yes, dinner matters, folks—more than you think.

First things first, let's talk about dinner's impact on sleep. You may think, "Hey, I can eat anything and still sleep like a baby!" But what you don't realize is that your dinner choices are quietly working behind the scenes to either set you up for a restful night or sabotage your sweet dreams. Eating a heavy, spicy, or greasy meal right before bed might lead to indigestion, acid reflux, and the kind of tossing and turning that makes you feel like you're trying to sleep on a roller coaster. And let's not even mention the dreaded midnight snack attack when your body suddenly craves something salty or sweet, turning your peaceful sleep into a food-fueled mission.

On the flip side, a light and balanced dinner can be your ticket to blissful sleep. A well-timed, nutritious meal helps to regulate your blood sugar levels, support digestion, and even produce those sleep-promoting hormones like melatonin. So, while that late-night pizza might be calling your name, think twice. Your sleep and morning grogginess will thank you later.

Now, let's talk personalization. Just like you wouldn't wear the same outfit to every occasion (unless you're a fashion rebel, in which case, power to you), dinner needs to be tailored to your lifestyle and body. Are you an athlete running marathons or someone who simply runs on caffeine and optimism? Your dinner should reflect that. If you're active, your body needs extra fuel to recover from those intense workouts. Protein-rich foods, whole grains, and healthy fats will keep you energized and help with muscle repair. But if you're more of a couch potato (no judgment here—we all love a good binge-watch), a light dinner with veggies and lean protein might be your best bet to avoid feeling sluggish the next morning.

The key to a perfect dinner? It's not about deprivation or indulgence, but finding the sweet spot—one that satisfies your hunger, nourishes your body, and doesn't leave you with a food coma. Dinner is your opportunity to show your body some love by providing it with the nutrients it needs to wind down and recharge for the next day. So, the next time you sit down to your evening meal, think of it as the grand finale to your day—a thoughtful, nourishing, and sleep-friendly ending to your daily food journey.

Early Dinner – Why It's a Game-Changer

Let's talk about early dinners. We've all been there—rushing home from work or getting through an evening of activities, only to find ourselves diving into a hefty meal at 9 p.m. But what if we told you that eating earlier in the evening could be your secret weapon for feeling better, sleeping better, and even looking better? Yes, that's right—an early dinner is like the underdog of meal timing, quietly working wonders while you're enjoying your post-dinner dessert (we won't judge, but maybe consider swapping it for fruit).

Benefits of Eating Early

Digestive Benefits: Imagine this: You eat an early dinner, your body has a few hours to process the meal, and by the time you hit the hay, your digestive system isn't still working overtime. Instead, it's relaxed, and you're cruising through a peaceful night's sleep. Eating late—especially a heavy meal—throws your digestive system into overdrive, leaving you feeling bloated, uncomfortable, and vaguely regretting every life choice that led to you eating that half-pizza, half-burger monstrosity at 10 p.m. Early dinners allow your stomach to start digesting while you're still awake, so it's not scrambling for hours to process that last-minute snack before bedtime.

Sleep Quality: If you've ever eaten a massive dinner right before bed, you know what comes next: restless tossing, turning, and generally cursing yourself for that second helping of pasta. Eating too late can disrupt your circadian rhythm (aka, the body's internal clock), which can affect your sleep quality. On the flip side, an early dinner, ideally consumed at least 2-3 hours before bedtime, gives your body a fighting chance to wind down. Your metabolism slows down as the evening progresses, so when you eat early, you allow your body to focus on relaxation, rather than frantically processing food as you try to drift off into dreamland. It's like giving your body permission to chill out and not race against time to burn through a massive meal.

Weight Management: You know those nights when you have a late dinner and then find yourself snacking mindlessly in the kitchen an hour later? Well, that's not helping your weight management goals. Eating earlier helps regulate your hunger hormones and supports metabolism, making it easier to control those late-night cravings. Plus, when you eat early, you're giving your body enough time to digest and burn off the calories before you hit the sack, making your weight management game stronger. If you've ever tried to sleep on a full stomach, you know that it's the recipe for a rough night. So, skipping that extra helping of mashed potatoes at midnight can actually work wonders on your waistline. Early dinners mean your body has time to digest the nutrients and actually use them, instead of storing them in all the wrong places.

What an Early Dinner Should Consist Of

Now that you're convinced that an early dinner is your golden ticket to feeling great, let's talk about what your plate should actually look like. An early dinner doesn't mean you should just eat a salad the size of your face or only snack on carrot sticks (unless that's your vibe, in which case, more power to you). The key is balance, my friend. We're not asking for a 10-course gourmet meal, just a sensible plate that will leave you feeling satisfied without sending you into a food coma.

Balanced Meal: A balanced dinner should include a combination of lean proteins (like chicken, tofu, or fish), healthy fats (think avocado, olive oil, or nuts), and fiber-rich vegetables (hello, broccoli, spinach, and peppers!). This combo will provide the fuel your body needs without overwhelming it. Lean protein helps repair muscles and keeps you feeling full. Healthy fats are like the superhero sidekicks that help with nutrient absorption and keep you satisfied for longer. And fiber-rich veggies? Well, they're the unsung heroes of digestion, helping things move smoothly while also being packed with vitamins and minerals.

Portion Control: Here's the thing: Your dinner doesn't need to be bigger than your lunch (we know, this sounds like blasphemy). In fact, smaller portions at dinner work wonders. Eating less at night reduces the chance of overeating or consuming excess calories that will be stored rather than used. Think of dinner as the closing act of the day—don't make it a 3-hour Broadway show. Keep portions moderate so your body isn't burdened with digesting a three-course meal while you're trying to relax. Your body is winding down for the night, and the last thing it needs is to spend hours working through an excessive meal.

Avoiding Heavy, Hard-to-Digest Foods: A burger with fries at 8 p.m. sounds tempting, right? It's comforting, delicious, and oh-so-satisfying. But here's the thing: Heavy, greasy, or spicy foods are not exactly a great choice for dinner. Sure, they may taste good in the moment, but your digestive system will curse you later. Fried foods, excessive sugar, and carbs in large amounts can make you feel bloated, sluggish, and downright uncomfortable when you hit the pillow. Instead, opt for meals that are light on your stomach but still packed with flavor. Grilled or baked chicken, roasted vegetables, quinoa, and a side of leafy greens are the real MVPs of dinner. They're easy on the stomach and won't make you feel like you swallowed a rock before trying to sleep.

Practical Tips for Scheduling an Early Dinner

So, how do you pull off an early dinner when the world (or your work schedule) is conspiring against you? No need to panic — we've got you covered. The key is to adapt your lifestyle and plan ahead.

- **Meal Prepping:** Planning ahead is your secret weapon. If you know you're going to be rushed in the evening, prep your meals in advance. It's the 21st century version of having your dinner ready to go at the perfect time. Make enough for a couple of days so you don't have to worry about cooking at 8 p.m. when you're ready to collapse from exhaustion. Plus, meal prepping means you can control portion sizes and ensure your meals are balanced and nutritious.
- **Having a Lighter Lunch:** If you want to make sure you're hungry for an early dinner, try having a lighter lunch. A big, heavy lunch can make you feel stuffed and less likely to want a smaller, lighter dinner. So, keep lunch on the lighter side

with salads, lean proteins, and some whole grains to make sure you're ready to eat earlier in the evening.

Personalized Dinners – Tailoring Meals to Your Needs

Let's face it—no two people are the same, so why should your dinner be a one-size-fits-all situation? Imagine walking into a restaurant and ordering the same meal as your friend. Sure, you both need food, but are you both going to feel satisfied, energized, and ready to conquer the world afterward? Probably not. Just like your body has unique needs throughout the day, your dinner should be tailored to those needs as well. So, let's dive into the art of personalizing your evening meal, making sure it works for *you*, no one else.

Recognizing Your Body's Needs

Your body is a finely tuned machine (even if it sometimes feels more like a rusty scooter), and understanding what it needs at dinner can mean the difference between feeling sluggish or waking up ready to tackle the world. Let's break down some of the most common body types, lifestyles, and activity levels to figure out what your personalized dinner should look like.

Different Body Types, Lifestyles, and Activity Levels

Let's start with the basics: Are you a marathon runner or a Netflix marathoner? Active individuals have very different needs than someone who's been sedentary all day (like that friend who, well, prefers their couch). If you're the athletic type, you need a dinner that helps repair muscles and refuel your body, while the more sedentary crowd should focus on meals that provide energy without overloading their system.

- **Active Individuals:** If you've been sweating it out in the gym, running around for hours, or chasing after kids, your body needs some serious recovery fuel. That means focusing on high-protein meals with healthy fats to repair muscles and moderate carbs to replenish glycogen stores. Think grilled chicken with quinoa and a side of sautéed spinach. Or maybe a tofu stir-fry with broccoli and sweet potatoes — something that gives your body the nutrients it craves after hours of activity. You want your dinner to be filling but not a food coma in a bowl. You don't want to be curled up on the couch groaning about your heavy meal right after a workout, right?

- **Sedentary Individuals:** For those of us who may have spent the day binge-watching the latest true-crime series (no judgment, we've all been there), your body doesn't need the same heavy carb load. Instead, opt for lighter meals that provide sustenance without causing a food coma. A lean protein, some roasted vegetables, and a small portion of healthy carbs (hello, quinoa) are the perfect balance. That way, your body isn't left with excess fuel it has nowhere to burn, and you won't feel sluggish as you wind down for bed.

Dinner for Mental Clarity

It's not just about your body's physical needs — dinner can also be the secret weapon for your mental clarity. That's right, folks, dinner can fuel your brain for the next day. Want to be sharp, focused, and ready to take on the world (or at least finish that to-do list)? You need to choose foods that boost brain function.

For cognitive clarity, try meals rich in omega-3 fatty acids (like salmon), antioxidants (think colorful veggies), and B vitamins (which you can find in whole grains and leafy greens). Not only will your brain thank you in the morning, but you'll also feel like the sharpest tool in the shed the next day — ready to tackle meetings, assignments, or simply nail your grocery list without getting distracted.

So, next time you're making dinner, think about it as fueling both your body *and* your brain. A nice baked salmon with a side of avocado and roasted asparagus is a perfect choice for cognitive function—because who doesn't want to feel like a genius after a satisfying meal?

Nutrient Focus Based on Goals

Now, let's talk about the real question everyone asks themselves: "What am I trying to achieve with this dinner?" Whether you're aiming to shed a few pounds, bulk up, or just maintain your current form, your dinner should reflect your personal goals. After all, you wouldn't wear flip-flops to a wedding (unless it's a fashion statement), so why would you eat the same meal regardless of your goals?

Weight Loss: Low-Carb, High-Protein Meals with Lots of Vegetables

If weight loss is on your agenda, then dinner should be more about eating for satisfaction without overloading on calories. A low-carb, high-protein meal is your best bet. Protein helps you feel full for longer, so you won't be raiding the fridge an hour later. Add in some vegetables for fiber, vitamins, and minerals, and voilà— you've got the perfect weight-loss meal. A grilled chicken breast with steamed broccoli and a side of cauliflower rice is the type of dinner that keeps you feeling light yet satisfied. The best part? You don't have to worry about that bloated feeling that comes with a carb-heavy, greasy meal.

Muscle Gain: Higher-Protein Meals with Healthy Fats and Moderate Carbs

For those looking to pack on muscle, your dinner needs to be a little more substantial. You need a solid amount of protein to repair those muscles after a workout, along with some healthy fats and moderate carbs to keep your energy levels steady. Think steak (or plant-based protein if that's your thing), a sweet potato, and a side of roasted Brussels sprouts. The protein will give your muscles what they need to rebuild, while the healthy fats and carbs will give you the energy to do it all again tomorrow. It's like you're fueling up for a workout *and* recovery all in one go—like a performance-enhancing meal.

Maintenance: Balanced Meals with All Macronutrients in Moderation

Ah, the sweet spot—maintenance. You're not trying to lose weight, nor are you trying to bulk up. You just want to keep things steady. For maintenance, focus on a balanced meal that includes a little bit of everything: lean protein, complex carbs, healthy fats, and fiber-rich veggies. Think grilled fish with quinoa, a side of avocado, and a nice salad. This type of dinner keeps you full, nourished, and on track without overloading on any single macronutrient.

Mindful Eating: The Forgotten Art

And finally, let's talk about how you *actually* eat your dinner. Yes, we're going there—mindful eating. If you've been scarfing down dinner while scrolling through your phone or watching TV, you're not alone. But here's the thing: Mindless eating isn't just bad for digestion—it's bad for your relationship with food, too. By paying attention to what you're eating and savoring each bite, you can actually help your body digest better, feel more satisfied, and avoid overeating.

Take your time, chew your food, and pay attention to how your body feels while you eat. Your stomach will thank you later, and you might even realize that you're full before you reach for that second helping. Bonus: Mindful eating helps you tune into your body's signals, so you can truly understand when you're hungry, when you're full, and when you just need a little something sweet for dessert.

The Importance of a Light Dinner

Ah, dinner—the final act of your day, the grand finale before you slip into the cozy embrace of your bed. It's that time when you gather around the table (or the couch, let's be real) to fill your belly and satisfy your taste buds. But here's the catch: It's *really* important that dinner isn't the food equivalent of a heavyweight champion. The secret to a peaceful night's sleep and waking up feeling like you actually got rest lies in making your dinner light, balanced, and easy on your system. Think of it as giving your stomach a warm hug, not a full-on wrestling match.

Why Lighter Meals Promote Better Sleep

Let's start with the science bit (don't worry, we'll keep it light). After a long day of running around, your body is tired, and your digestive system is no exception. Imagine trying to fall asleep with a heavy, greasy meal still lingering in your stomach—your body's doing backflips trying to digest all that food, while you're just trying to get some shut-eye. This is where light dinners come in like a hero in a rom-com: They help you fall asleep faster, avoid digestive drama, and let you wake up feeling like you actually *slept*.

When you eat a heavy meal, your body works overtime trying to digest all that food. This can lead to acid reflux, bloating, and just general discomfort—like your stomach's having a party without you. Instead of zoning out in front of your favorite show or doing a little pre-sleep reading, you're clutching your belly and wondering why your dinner has turned against you. Plus, the more you eat, the harder your body has to work to process the food. This puts your body in overdrive when it should be winding down.

On the flip side, a light, well-balanced dinner works wonders for a good night's sleep. By eating something easy to digest, your body isn't scrambling to break down a four-course meal while you're trying to dream about tropical vacations. Instead, a light dinner allows your digestive system to rest and do its job without making you feel like you're in the middle of a digestive triathlon. As a result, you wake up refreshed, ready to take on the day — without that 'food coma' fog hanging over your head.

Ideal Foods for a Light Dinner

Now that we know why a lighter dinner is the key to a blissful night of sleep, let's talk about what foods should be on your plate. Don't worry, light doesn't mean *boring*. You can still enjoy delicious, satisfying meals without feeling like you're eating a salad and calling it a day. Here are some great options:

High-Protein, Low-Carb Options Lean proteins are your best friend for a light dinner. They're easy to digest, don't weigh you down, and help keep you full without piling on the calories. Think chicken breast, fish, turkey, or tofu if you're plant-based. These protein sources are like the reliable sidekick of your meal — helping you stay satisfied but not giving you that "I need to roll myself into bed" feeling. A piece of grilled chicken with a side of roasted veggies? Perfect. Baked fish with some steamed broccoli? Even better. Or if you're in the mood for something plant-based, throw together a tofu stir-fry with your favorite greens — simple, light, and delicious.

Vegetables Ah, vegetables — nature's way of saying, "Here, have something that won't make your stomach mad." You can't go wrong with leafy greens, cauliflower rice, or roasted vegetables. Leafy greens like spinach, kale, or arugula are full of fiber and vitamins, and they're light enough not to weigh you down. Plus, they're like the cool sidekick in your dinner story — they play nice with pretty much everything! Roasted cauliflower rice, anyone? It's the trendy alternative to regular rice and won't leave you feeling bloated. Roasting veggies like zucchini, bell peppers, or Brussels sprouts adds a little crunch and flavor to your plate, without the digestive drama. Vegetables are like the peaceful zen garden your stomach has always wanted.

Healthy Fats: You didn't think we'd leave you hanging with just protein and veggies, did you? Healthy fats are an essential part of a well-rounded, light dinner. Think avocados, nuts, olive oil — foods that nourish your body without being too heavy. Add some slices of avocado to your salad or drizzle olive oil on your veggies before roasting them. If you're feeling a little snacky, grab a handful of almonds or walnuts — packed with healthy fats that are gentle on your digestion. These fats help keep you satisfied and don't overload your system, so you can get that good sleep you've been dreaming about.

What to Avoid: Now, let's get real for a second. There are certain foods you should *definitely* steer clear of if you want to avoid sleepless nights and a belly full of regret. While you might crave that cheesy pasta or a huge steak at the end of a long day, those heavy foods can sabotage your sleep in ways that make you want to weep into your pillow.

Spicy or Rich Foods: Let's start with the obvious: spicy foods. Sure, they're delicious, but they can leave you with heartburn or indigestion, and we're not here for that drama. The last thing you want while you're trying to sleep is your stomach doing the cha-cha with the ghost of last night's chili. And rich, creamy dishes? They might sound appealing, but they're often a lot for your digestive system to handle. Your stomach will be working overtime to break down all that heavy food, and you'll be left tossing and turning while your body plays catch-up.

Excessive Caffeine, Sugar, or Alcohol: We know, we know — your evening routine might involve a little bit of sugar or a glass of wine. But, and here's the kicker, those aren't exactly conducive to good sleep. Caffeine, especially in the evening, can leave you wide awake at 3 a.m. wondering why you agreed to that cup of coffee after dinner. Sugar can send your blood sugar levels on a rollercoaster ride, leaving you wired and restless. Alcohol, while it might make you feel sleepy at first, can disrupt your sleep cycle and leave you feeling groggy the next morning. So, try to skip the sugary snacks, caffeine bombs, and nightcaps if you want to wake up feeling like you've actually slept.

How Light Doesn't Mean Bland

You might be thinking, "Okay, so I need to eat light—does that mean I'm stuck with bland, tasteless food?" Absolutely not. Just because you're keeping things light doesn't mean you have to sacrifice flavor. The secret? Herbs and spices.

You can easily transform a light dinner into a flavor-packed meal with a few key ingredients. Add some fresh basil to your grilled chicken, sprinkle a little cumin and paprika on your roasted veggies, or drizzle a dash of lemon juice over your tofu stir-fry. Spices like turmeric, ginger, garlic, and cinnamon not only add flavor but come with a host of health benefits. So don't be afraid to get creative with your seasoning. Your taste buds—and your digestive system—will thank you.

The Link Between Dinner and Sleep Quality

Ah, the eternal struggle: you want to eat dinner, but you also want to fall asleep without the terrifying idea of tossing and turning all night. So, what's the deal? Why does eating a late-night snack sometimes feel like an invitation to your body to turn into a restless, sleepless, hangry monster? Well, my friend, let's take a look at how your dinner might be sneaking up and sabotaging your beauty sleep—and what you can do to make sure your dinner is working in your favor.

How Late Meals Mess With Your Sleep

It's 9:30 p.m., you've just finished that last meeting, and you're suddenly *hungry*. And by hungry, we mean more than a snack. Your stomach's doing the Macarena, and you're convinced that a pizza is the only solution to your late-night woes. But here's the thing—eating too close to bedtime is like inviting your digestive system to a midnight rave when it's supposed to be getting some shut-eye. Let me explain.

The human body runs on a biological clock, also known as the circadian rhythm, which is like the master scheduler of your entire existence. This little clock dictates when you should wake up, when you should eat, and—very importantly—when you should sleep. When you eat late, you're throwing a wrench into the whole sleep process. Your body needs time to digest, and by eating late, you're forcing your body to multitask: digesting food and trying to wind down. It's like trying to run a marathon while balancing a stack of books—you're not going to win any medals.

But it gets worse. When you eat a big meal right before bed, your body has to produce extra stomach acid to break down that food, and this can mess with your sleep. You might wake up feeling like you swallowed a rock, with indigestion or acid reflux keeping you up all night. Not exactly the recipe for waking up feeling rested and ready to take on the world, is it?

The Science Behind Late Meals and Melatonin

Now let's get a little *science-y* (don't worry, we'll keep it fun). When you eat late, it messes with your body's ability to produce melatonin, the hormone that signals your body to fall asleep. Melatonin is like the gentle lullaby your brain sings to itself, saying, "Hey, it's time to relax and hit the hay." But, and here's the kicker, your digestive system needs a little time to finish up its work. If you've just eaten a burger and fries (or, you know, a pizza), your body is busy processing all that while trying to get you to sleep.

The result? You end up lying there staring at the ceiling while your body tries to figure out if it's time to sleep or run a marathon.

In short, eating too late can make melatonin production trickier. And without melatonin, well, you're left struggling to fall asleep, with your brain in full "I'll just check Instagram for five minutes" mode, until the sun starts peeking out the window. So, as much as that late-night snack might seem tempting, your body would prefer to finish its digestive duties a little earlier in the evening.

What to Eat to Promote Restful Sleep

Here's the fun part: you can eat food that helps you sleep! Yep, that's right. There's a whole world of delicious foods that promote melatonin and serotonin production (those are the sleep and happiness hormones, by the way), without keeping you up all night thinking about your to-do list. You don't need to raid the kitchen for junk food or sugary snacks; there are healthier, sleep-friendly options that won't make you feel like a bloated balloon.

Foods that Promote Melatonin and Serotonin

1. Almonds: Not just a fancy snack. These little nuts are packed with magnesium, which helps your muscles relax. They're also rich in melatonin, so eating a handful before bed is like giving your body a signal that it's time to unwind. Plus, they're delicious, so no excuses!

2. Bananas: Ah, the humble banana. This potassium-packed fruit can help regulate your blood sugar levels, keeping you from waking up in the middle of the night looking for a midnight snack. They also contain tryptophan (yep, the same compound in turkey that makes you feel like napping after Thanksgiving), which boosts serotonin production. Translation: They make you sleepy, in the best way.

3. Turkey: Yes, your Thanksgiving hero has a trick or two up its sleeve. Turkey is a great source of tryptophan, which helps

your body produce serotonin, the "feel-good" hormone that leads to better sleep. So, maybe save the turkey for dinner instead of leaving it just for holidays.

4. Kiwi: You might look at this fuzzy little fruit and think, "What kind of sorcery is this?" But kiwi has been shown to improve sleep quality. It contains antioxidants and serotonin, both of which help regulate your sleep-wake cycle. Have a couple of these before bed, and you'll be dreaming of unicorns in no time.

5. Cherries: Cherries are a natural source of melatonin, which is exactly what you need to encourage a peaceful slumber. Plus, they're sweet and juicy, so you'll be like, "This is a snack I can get behind."

Herbal Teas: Your New Best Friend

If you're someone who needs a warm, comforting drink to wind down, look no further than herbal teas. Chamomile, peppermint, and lavender are the stars of the tea world when it comes to promoting sleep. These herbs have natural sedative properties that can help your mind relax and prepare for sleep. Brew yourself a cozy cup of chamomile tea, and let the gentle sleep magic begin.

1. Chamomile: This is the classic sleep-friendly tea. It's been used for centuries as a natural remedy for insomnia. Chamomile calms the nervous system, helping you drift off to sleep more easily.

2. Peppermint: If you've had a big meal and your stomach is still doing cartwheels, peppermint tea can help soothe digestion and promote relaxation. Plus, the cool, refreshing taste is perfect after a hearty meal.

3. Lavender: Lavender is well-known for its relaxing properties. Drinking a warm cup of lavender tea can send your body the message that it's time to relax and wind down for the night.

Timing of Your Dinner: The Optimal Window for Eating

This might sound like a no-brainer, but timing really is everything. You've probably heard the age-old rule: Don't eat too close to bedtime. And here's why: your body needs time to digest, and if you're eating dinner right before crashing, your body's doing a bit of overtime to process all that food, making it harder for you to fall asleep.

The general recommendation is to aim to eat dinner about 2-3 hours before heading to bed. This allows your body to complete most of its digestion and start winding down. That way, when you lie down, your body isn't racing to break down a large meal and you can slip into a deeper, more restful sleep.

Midnight Cravings – The Dos and Don'ts

Ah, midnight cravings. The sneaky little gremlins that show up when you've just drifted off to sleep, or maybe you're lying in bed scrolling through TikTok, when suddenly your brain whispers, "Hey, you deserve a snack." It's like your stomach has decided to become the villain in your sleep saga, right when you're about to peacefully drift off. So why do these cravings strike, and how can you deal with them without derailing your entire sleep (and diet) routine?

The Common Struggle: Why Midnight Cravings Happen

It's not just your willpower that's at fault when the 3 a.m. hunger pangs hit. In fact, midnight cravings often have more to do with your hormones than with your lack of self-control. Cortisol, the stress hormone, can spike in the evening, triggering feelings of hunger. Meanwhile, another hormone, ghrelin (your "hunger hormone"), might decide to party just as you're trying to get some shut-eye, sending your brain a message that you NEED food — like, right now.

Then there's the emotional side of things. Have you ever had a tough day, only to find yourself craving comfort food late at night? That's because your body associates food with comfort. Combine stress, habit, and boredom, and you've got a recipe for a late-night snack attack.

Why Giving In to Midnight Snacks is a Bad Idea

Alright, now let's talk about why giving in to these cravings isn't exactly winning you any sleep prizes. For starters, eating too late can interfere with your digestive system. When you snack late, your body is still working hard to digest food while you're trying to sleep. This not only affects your sleep quality but also leads to that *lovely* feeling of indigestion or acid reflux in the middle of the night. Not exactly the sweet dreams you were hoping for, right?

Let's not forget that eating at night can lead to unwanted weight gain. Studies show that late-night eating disrupts your metabolism, and when your body doesn't burn off those late-night calories, they're stored as fat. So, that midnight bowl of ice cream? It's not doing your waistline (or your sleep) any favors.

Healthy Alternatives for Midnight Cravings

Now, I'm not here to ruin your fun. If you absolutely must satisfy your midnight cravings, let's make it count. There are healthier options that won't derail your entire day's worth of eating, and they won't leave you awake at 3 a.m. regretting your life choices.

1. A small handful of nuts: Almonds or walnuts are a great option. They're full of magnesium, which helps relax your muscles and supports a good night's sleep. Plus, they're easy to munch on and won't leave you feeling bloated.

2. Yogurt with berries: It's light, easy to digest, and packed with probiotics that are great for your gut. Add some antioxidants with a handful of fresh berries, and you've got yourself a delicious snack that's also good for you.
3. A slice of turkey: You know that tryptophan everyone talks about when it comes to turkey? Well, it's real. Turkey helps produce serotonin and melatonin, which are your body's natural sleep aids. Just one slice and you're practically sleepwalking to dreamland.
4. Hydration: Sometimes, cravings aren't about hunger—they're about thirst. Drinking a glass of water or a warm cup of herbal tea (chamomile, anyone?) can help curb those cravings. Plus, it's a nice way to trick your brain into thinking it's snack time without the actual snacking.

When to Avoid Midnight Snacks

Okay, here's the trick: Not all hunger is *real* hunger. Sometimes it's just your body playing tricks on you. So, how do you know if your midnight craving is legitimate or just a temptation in disguise? One word: listen. Is your stomach growling because you genuinely didn't eat enough during the day, or is it just your mind trying to justify that extra scoop of peanut butter?

If you're sure it's *true* hunger, a healthy snack is your best bet. But if it's just a craving for something salty, sweet, or sinful, it's time to *resist*. Trust me, your future self (and your waistline) will thank you. If you don't really need the food, why bother? Your body needs rest, not a midnight buffet.

The Evening Meal – A Thoughtful and Balanced End to Your Day

So, here we are, at the end of our dinner journey—let's wrap things up with a healthy dose of common sense (and maybe a little bit of humor because, hey, we've all been there). Dinner isn't just another meal you rush through while half-watching your favorite TV show. Nope. It's the grand finale of your day, and it deserves to be treated like a five-star performance. In fact, if dinner were a movie, it would be the one that sets the tone for your whole night. The right dinner doesn't just fill you up, it sets you up for sleep, boosts your energy, and helps maintain that beautiful balance we all need.

Early, Light, and Tailored to You

Now, let's recap. Eating early (like, before your stomach starts complaining at midnight) is your ticket to better digestion and, yes, a better sleep. Give your body the time it needs to properly digest your meal and prepare for rest. But don't get carried away with a five-course meal! Keep things light—your body will thank you, especially when it's time to hit the hay. And remember, dinner should be personalized. Whether you're an athlete in need of extra protein or just trying to shed a couple of pounds, dinner should work for you, not against you. A lean protein, some veggies, and a drizzle of healthy fat can go a long way to keep you full without feeling like you're going to burst into flames halfway through your Netflix binge.

Dinner is a Big Deal—Don't Treat It Like an Afterthought!

And let's not forget, a good dinner has the power to set your entire mood for the night. If you eat a huge meal right before bed, chances are you'll wake up feeling bloated and cranky, and trust me, that's no way to start a productive day. However, if you've made sure to eat the right things at the right time, your body will be ready to unwind and restore itself for the next day. Your sleep quality will improve, you won't be tossing and turning, and you'll probably wake up feeling like you've conquered the world—well, maybe not the world, but at least your morning cup of coffee won't feel like a lifeline.

The Takeaway? Make Dinner Work for You!

Here's the final golden nugget of wisdom: dinner is not the time for mindless eating. It's not a place for mindless snacking or indulging in foods that'll have you up all night regretting your choices. It's your opportunity to nourish your body, to fuel it properly for the night ahead. Make dinner work for you by keeping it balanced, light, and aligned with your goals. Want better sleep? Have a lighter meal. Want to stay on top of your health game? Keep it personalized. Want to wake up in a good mood instead of clutching your stomach in the morning? Avoid those heavy, greasy meals that make you feel like you've eaten a brick.

In the end, dinner doesn't have to be complicated. With a little thought and effort, it can be a wonderful way to nourish your body, recharge your energy, and prepare yourself for a restful night. So, next time you sit down for dinner, remember that it's more than just "the last meal of the day." It's the key to feeling good, sleeping well, and waking up ready to take on whatever comes next. Bon appétit!

Carbs: The Good, The Bad, and the Delicious

Carbohydrates. Just the word alone can spark heated debates in fitness circles, dietary forums, and even between best friends deciding where to eat. One moment, carbs are our best friends (hello, warm, buttery bread), and the next, they're public enemy number one (goodbye, pasta — again?). But let's set the record straight: carbs are not the villain in your health journey. When consumed correctly, they can be your ultimate energy source, brain booster, and mood stabilizer.

Think of carbohydrates as the body's primary source of fuel, much like gasoline for your car. They come in three main forms:

1. Simple Carbs – These are the sprinters of the carb world. They provide quick bursts of energy but don't last long. Found in sugar, soda, candy, and white bread, they're the reason your energy crashes faster than a toddler post-birthday party.
2. Complex Carbs – The marathon runners. These take longer to digest, keeping you full and energized for hours. Whole grains, legumes, and vegetables fall into this category.
3. Fiber – The unsung hero of carbs. Fiber isn't digested like the other two but helps regulate blood sugar, aids digestion, and keeps things… moving along smoothly, if you catch my drift.

Why Are Carbs Important?

Ah, carbohydrates — the misunderstood hero of nutrition. One day they're the enemy, the next they're being praised as a gym-goer's best friend, of course for muscle building. But the truth is, carbs do a lot more than just make food taste amazing (though, let's be honest, they satiate your soul, therefore, that makes them addictive). They're an essential part of a balanced diet and play a crucial role in keeping your body running smoothly.

So before you swear off bread forever, let's talk about why carbs actually deserve a spot on your plate.

1. Energy Production: The Body's Favorite Fuel

Carbs are the fuel that keeps your body's engine running. When you eat them, they break down into glucose, powering everything from your muscles to your brain.

Ever tried skipping carbs and then wondered why you feel sluggish, irritable, and as drained as a phone stuck at 1% — especially if you have an active lifestyle? That's because carbs provide fast, efficient energy, which is why athletes and highly active individuals rely on them to perform at their best.

However, not all carbs are created equal. Overconsumption or choosing the wrong types can lead to energy crashes, weight gain, and metabolic imbalances. Carbs work best when paired with other nutrients like fiber, protein, and healthy fats, ensuring sustained energy and better digestion.

The real issue isn't carbs themselves — it's how they're consumed. Rather than being the villain, carbs are a key player in a balanced diet, providing the energy your body needs to thrive.

2. Brain Function: Because Thinking Requires Fuel Too

Your brain may not be lifting weights or running marathons, but it's one of the biggest consumers of glucose. It runs on sugar the way a sports car runs on premium fuel. In fact, your brain alone uses about 20% of your body's energy each day.

Ever noticed how hard it is to focus when you're hungry? Or why low-carb diets sometimes leave people feeling foggy and forgetful?

That's because when your glucose levels drop, so does your brainpower. Suddenly, simple decisions feel impossible, and you might even forget why you walked into a room in the first place.

A steady supply of good carbs—like whole grains, fruits, and veggies—keeps your brain sharp, helping you think clearly and stay productive.

3. Mood Regulation: Why You Crave Cookies When You're Stressed

Carbs don't just fuel your body; they also have a direct impact on your mood. They help produce serotonin, the "feel-good" hormone responsible for keeping you happy and relaxed which often makes you emotionally dependent on them.

This explains why you instinctively reach for a bowl of pasta, a slice of pizza, or a warm chocolate chip cookie when life gets stressful. However, it's important to distinguish between your body's natural need for carbs and emotional eating patterns. While we're here to celebrate carbs as the energy-giving hero, mindful consumption is key. Choosing the right carbs in the right amounts ensures you get their benefits without becoming overly dependent on them for emotional comfort.

Of course, not all carbs are created equal—while a sugar binge might give you a temporary mood boost, it's best to opt for complex carbs like sweet potatoes, quinoa, millets, wholegrains and legumes for a steady, long-lasting supply of serotonin-boosting goodness.

4. Muscle Recovery: Carbs and Gains Go Hand-in-Hand

After a workout, your muscles are like a sponge, ready to soak up glycogen (the stored form of carbs) to repair and rebuild.

Skipping post-workout carbs is like trying to refill an empty gas tank with just air. Sure, protein helps with muscle repair, but without carbs, your recovery will be slow, and you'll feel sore for much longer.

This is why athletes make sure to refuel with a mix of protein *and* carbs after exercise—because muscles need both to grow and recover effectively.

When is the Best Time to Eat Carbs?

Ah, carbs—our delicious, doughy, and sometimes controversial friends. While they're essential for energy, brain function, and overall well-being, *when* you eat them can make a big difference in how they affect your body. You wouldn't chug an espresso at midnight (hopefully), so why treat carbs any differently? Let's break down the best times to fuel up and when to ease off the gas.

Pre-Workout: Fuel Up for Performance

Ever tried working out on an empty stomach? It's like trying to drive a car with no gas—you won't get very far. Your muscles need a quick energy source, and carbs provide that instant boost so you can power through your workout without running on fumes.

Best choices (30-60 minutes before exercise):

- A banana (nature's perfect pre-workout snack!)
- A protein smoothie with dates
- A handful of trail mix

These snacks give you the fast-digesting energy needed to crush your gym session without feeling sluggish.

Post-Workout: Refill the Tank

After a tough workout, your muscles are basically screaming, "Feed me!" This is the prime time to consume carbs because your body is in absorption mode, ready to soak up glycogen to repair and rebuild.

Best choices (within 30-60 minutes post-workout):
- Sweet potatoes with grilled chicken
- Brown rice with lean protein
- Quinoa salad with veggies
- Protein smoothie loaded with fiber

Pairing carbs with protein helps maximize muscle repair and ensures you won't wake up feeling like you got hit by a truck.

Lunch: The Main Show

Carbs are best enjoyed at the right time and in the right way. After fueling your body with protein and healthy fats to break your morning fast, lunch is the perfect window to introduce carbs — when your metabolism is at its peak and your body is ready to use them efficiently.

Power-Packed Lunch Carbs:

- Mix Veggie Fried Rice (paired with the desired portion of protein)
- Millet Roti & Stir-Fried Veggies
- Lentils & Quinoa Bowl
- Chickpea Rice Bowl

Elevate your meal with a side of fresh salad or yogurt for extra probiotics and fiber, making your carb intake even more nourishing and delicious!

Evening: The Great Carbs Debate

Carbs at night—yes or no? The internet is *raging* over this one, but here's the truth: you absolutely can eat carbs in the evening.

If you work out at night, your body needs carbs for recovery. Even if you don't, complex carbs can actually help you sleep better by increasing serotonin levels.

Best evening carbs (paired with the desired portion of protein):

- Lentil rice with salad for dinner
- A small serving of gluten free pasta loaded with veggies
- A baked sweet potato
- A warm bowl of quinoa porridge

The key? Avoid heavy, *sugary* carbs right before bed. You don't need a sugar rush when you're trying to wind down.

The Good, The Bad, and The Overly Processed

Carbs have been through *a lot*—from being hailed as the holy grail of energy to being demonized as the culprit behind weight gain. But the truth? Not all carbs are created equal. Some are nutritional powerhouses, while others are sneaky little troublemakers in disguise. Let's break it down:

The Good Carbs: Your Trusty Sidekicks

Good carbs are like that reliable friend who always shows up on time and remembers your birthday. They're packed with fiber, vitamins, and nutrients that keep your body happy and healthy.

Best sources of good carbs:

- Whole Grains: Rice, millets, quinoa, sourdough bread, and oats. They digest slowly, keeping you full longer and preventing that dreaded afternoon slump.
- Fruits and Vegetables: Apples, berries, carrots, and leafy greens come loaded with fiber, antioxidants, and natural sugars—no artificial nonsense here.
- Legumes: Beans, lentils, and chickpeas are *carb and protein hybrids*—giving you energy while keeping your muscles strong.

- Nuts and Seeds: While higher in fats, they also provide good-quality carbs, plus protein and fiber to keep your energy levels stable.

Good carbs don't just fuel your body—they *nourish* it. Think of them as the VIP section of the carb world.

The Bad Carbs: Proceed with Caution

These carbs aren't necessarily evil, but they're like that friend who means well but keeps giving you questionable advice. They offer quick energy but often lead to a crash, leaving you sluggish and craving more junk.

Carbs to be wary of:

- White Bread & White Pasta: They've been stripped of fiber and nutrients, making them digest *way* too fast. The result? Blood sugar spikes followed by a crash that leaves you hungrier than before.
- Sugary Cereals: They may *look* healthy with all those vitamins listed on the box, but if sugar is the first ingredient, it's basically dessert disguised as breakfast.
- Fruit Juices: Sounds healthy, right? Wrong. Most store-bought juices have as much sugar as soda, minus the fiber that makes whole fruit a better choice.

These carbs aren't completely off-limits, but they should be eaten in moderation—like cake at a birthday party, not cake for breakfast (*tempting, but no*).

The Overly Processed Carbs: The Trouble-Makers

Now, these guys? They're the ones who sweet-talk you into bad decisions. They taste amazing, but they offer zero nutritional value and can seriously mess with your metabolism over time.

Biggest offenders:

- Candy & Soda: Nothing but sugar, artificial flavors, and regret.
- Pastries & Chips: They're delicious, but packed with refined carbs and unhealthy fats.
- High-Fructose Corn Syrup Everything: Found in sodas, cereals, flavored yogurts, and even some "healthy" granola bars—this sneaky ingredient makes you crave more sugar, creating a vicious cycle.

These carbs should be treated like that toxic ex—fun in the moment but ultimately *not* good for you.

Carbs Aren't the Enemy

At the end of the day, carbs are essential, delicious, and, when chosen wisely, beneficial to your health. Instead of fearing them, focus on quality, timing, and balance. Eat the whole grains, savor the fruits, and yes, enjoy that occasional dessert—without the guilt trip!

After all, life's too short to skip the good stuff. Just maybe don't eat an entire cake before bed. (Unless it's your birthday. Then, all bets are off.)

Protein: The Mighty Macronutrient

If macronutrients had a popularity contest, carbs would be the fun, outgoing one everyone loves at parties, fats would be the misunderstood genius, and protein—well, protein would be the responsible one that keeps everything running smoothly. It's the backbone of muscle growth, the key to satiety, and the secret behind that post-workout glow. Despite what some diet trends might have you believe, protein isn't just for gym enthusiasts chugging protein shakes—it's essential for everyone. Whether you're looking to build strength, lose fat, or simply feel better overall, understanding protein's role in your body can be a game-changer.

So, let's break it down: why is protein so important, how much do you actually need, and what's the best way to get it? Get ready to dive into the world of amino acids, muscle repair, and food choices that will help you fuel your body the right way.

Why Is Protein Important?

Protein isn't just another nutrient on your plate—it's literally the building block of life. Every cell in your body, from your muscles and skin to your hair and organs, relies on protein to function properly. Without it, your body wouldn't be able to grow, repair, or maintain itself. But what exactly does protein do that makes it so crucial?

Protein and Muscle Repair

Ever felt sore after an intense workout? That's your muscles crying out for help. Exercise, especially strength training, causes small tears in muscle fibers. Protein comes to the rescue by repairing these tears, making your muscles stronger and more resilient over time. This is why athletes and fitness enthusiasts are so obsessed with their protein intake — it's their key to better recovery and improved performance.

But even if you don't lift weights or run marathons, your body still needs protein to maintain muscle mass. As we age, muscle naturally begins to break down (a process called sarcopenia). Eating enough protein helps slow down muscle loss and keeps you feeling strong and active well into old age.

Protein for Weight Management

Ever wondered why high-protein diets are often recommended for weight loss? It's simple: protein keeps you fuller for longer. Unlike carbs, which burn quickly and leave you craving snacks, protein takes longer to digest, reducing hunger and keeping cravings in check.

Additionally, protein has a high thermic effect — which means your body actually burns more calories digesting protein than it does with carbs or fats. So, by increasing your protein intake, you're not only staying full but also giving your metabolism a little boost which make protein a weapon to lose fat.

The Role of Protein in Overall Health

Protein isn't just about muscles and weight loss. It's essential for hormone production, immune function, and even brain health. Many of the body's most important hormones — like insulin, growth hormone, and even serotonin (the "feel-good" hormone) — are made up of proteins.

Have you ever noticed that when you're sick or recovering from an injury, doctors often recommend a protein-rich diet? That's because protein plays a major role in healing and immune defense. Your body needs amino acids (the building blocks of protein) to produce antibodies that fight infections.

So, whether you want strong muscles, better focus, glowing skin, or a stronger immune system, protein is your best friend.

How Much Protein Do You Actually Need?

The general guideline for protein consumption is based on body weight. For sedentary individuals, the recommended daily intake is 0.8g per kilogram of body weight. This is the minimum amount to prevent protein deficiency and support general bodily functions.

For those who are more physically active, protein needs increase to 1.2 to 2.0g per kilogram of body weight. This is especially important for individuals who engage in regular physical activity, such as walking, running, or cycling. The increase in protein helps to repair muscle tissues and replace the proteins that are broken down during exercise.

When it comes to athletes or individuals focused on muscle-building, the protein requirement becomes higher. To optimize muscle growth and recovery, the recommendation jumps to 1.6 to 2.2g per kilogram of body weight. This higher intake ensures that the body has enough amino acids to support muscle protein synthesis and promote the development of lean muscle mass.

Let's consider an individual weighing 70kg (154 lbs) who leads an active lifestyle. According to the recommendations, they should aim for 84g to 140g of protein per day, depending on the intensity and frequency of their physical activities. For someone looking to gain muscle, this number should be on the higher end of the scale.

The Best Sources of Protein

Animal-Based Protein Sources

Animal proteins are considered complete proteins, meaning they contain all nine essential amino acids that our bodies can't produce on their own. If you include animal products in your diet, these are some of the best sources:

- Eggs: Often regarded as one of the most nutrient-dense protein sources, eggs are a perfect balance of protein, fats, and vitamins. They're affordable, versatile, and can be included in various meals.
- Chicken & Turkey: These lean poultry options are packed with protein and low in fat, making them excellent choices for a healthy diet. Both are easy to incorporate into different cuisines and meal plans.
- Fish & Seafood: Rich in protein and omega-3 fatty acids, fish like salmon, tuna, and sardines are excellent for heart and brain health. Shellfish such as shrimp and lobster also offer protein along with minerals like zinc and iron.
- Beef & Lamb: While higher in fat, beef and lamb are excellent sources of protein and contain iron, which is vital for energy production. However, they should be consumed in moderation, especially if you're aiming for lean protein sources.
- Dairy Products: Dairy, such as Greek yogurt, cottage cheese, and milk, is packed with protein and calcium. Greek yogurt is also high in probiotics, which are beneficial for gut health.

Plant-Based Protein Sources

For those following a vegetarian or vegan diet, there are plenty of plant-based options to meet your protein needs. Most plant proteins are incomplete, meaning they lack one or more essential amino acids, but by combining different sources, you can still get all the necessary proteins.

- Lentils & Beans: High in both protein and fiber, these legumes are a filling and affordable way to get plant-based protein. They can be added to soups, salads, and stews.
- Chickpeas & Hummus: Chickpeas, whether used in salads, stews, or made into hummus, provide a great protein boost. Hummus is a tasty and versatile spread that can be enjoyed with veggies, bread, or crackers.
- Tofu & Tempeh: Both made from soybeans, tofu and tempeh are excellent protein sources. They absorb flavors well and can be used in various dishes, from stir-fries to curries.
- Quinoa: Unlike many plant-based proteins, quinoa is a complete protein, meaning it contains all nine essential amino acids. It's also rich in fiber and easy to cook.
- Nuts & Seeds: Almonds, chia seeds, flaxseeds, and other nuts and seeds are great for snacking or adding to smoothies. They provide a protein boost along with healthy fats and fiber.

When Is the Best Time to Eat Protein?

Protein timing can be just as important as the total amount you consume, especially if you're working towards specific goals like muscle gain, weight loss, or improving overall energy. While it's essential to spread protein intake evenly throughout the day, certain times of the day can offer additional benefits depending on your objectives. Here's a breakdown of the best times to eat protein to maximize its effects.

1. Breakfast: Start Strong

Starting your day with a protein-rich breakfast sets the tone for your metabolism and helps stabilize blood sugar levels. A breakfast that's high in protein, such as eggs, Greek yogurt, or a protein smoothie, will provide sustained energy throughout the morning. This is a much better option than carb-heavy breakfasts (like sugary cereals or white bread), which tend to lead to a spike in blood sugar followed by a crash, leaving you feeling hungry and fatigued before mid-morning. Protein is digested more slowly than carbs, meaning it helps keep you fuller longer and curbs mid-morning cravings.

Including protein in the morning is also beneficial for your muscles, especially if you are active. Consuming protein early in the day helps kickstart muscle protein synthesis — the process by which your body builds and repairs muscle. This can be especially important if you're aiming for muscle maintenance or growth. A breakfast packed with protein can ensure you're setting a solid foundation for the rest of the day, supporting both muscle health and energy levels.

2. Pre-Workout Protein: Fuel for Performance

Before hitting the gym or engaging in any strenuous physical activity, eating a small meal containing both protein and carbohydrates can help fuel your body. Carbohydrates provide immediate energy, while protein supports muscle preservation. Eating protein before a workout helps prevent muscle breakdown during exercise and ensures that your muscles have amino acids available for repair and growth as you exercise.

A pre-workout meal doesn't need to be heavy — something light and easily digestible is best. Examples of good pre-workout protein sources include a banana with peanut butter, a small protein smoothie, or a handful of nuts and seeds. The combination of protein and carbs gives your body the energy it needs for performance while reducing the risk of muscle loss during physical exertion.

Having protein before a workout also helps stabilize your blood sugar levels and prevents dips in energy. This can improve your workout performance and endurance, especially for longer or more intense training sessions.

3. Post-Workout Protein: The Recovery Window

After a workout, your muscles are particularly sensitive to nutrient intake, and the 30–60 minute window following exercise is often referred to as the "recovery window." During this period, your muscles are primed to absorb nutrients that aid in the repair and rebuilding process. This is the ideal time to consume protein, as it helps repair muscle fibers that have been broken down during exercise.

Post-workout protein intake is crucial for muscle recovery. It promotes muscle protein synthesis, reducing muscle soreness and aiding in faster recovery. Whey protein is one of the most popular choices after a workout due to its quick digestibility, but other sources like chicken, fish, or a protein shake also work well. If you pair protein with a small amount of carbohydrates, you can also replenish glycogen stores that were depleted during your workout. The ideal post-workout meal is one that contains about 10-20g of protein along with 30-40g of carbohydrates to optimize recovery.

This post-workout period is key for maximizing the results of your exercise routine. Without sufficient protein intake after a workout, you may experience slower recovery times and less progress toward muscle-building goals.

4. Protein Before Bed: Muscle Maintenance

Eating protein before bed can help prevent muscle breakdown during the night, especially when you're sleeping for several hours without food. A slow-digesting protein source, like casein protein or cottage cheese, is perfect for this. These proteins digest slowly and provide a steady release of amino acids to your muscles throughout the night, which helps maintain muscle mass while you sleep. This is especially beneficial for individuals looking to build muscle or prevent muscle loss while in a calorie deficit for weight loss.

Casein, in particular, is a great option because it forms a gel in the stomach that slows digestion, meaning your body continues to receive a steady stream of protein even as you rest. If you prefer a whole food option, cottage cheese is an excellent choice because it's high in casein and packed with other nutrients, including calcium and probiotics.

Having protein before bed not only helps with muscle recovery but also supports overall metabolic health. Plus, it can keep you from waking up feeling hungry in the morning, as the slow digestion of protein keeps you feeling satiated throughout the night.

To maximize protein's benefits for muscle recovery, energy, and overall health, it's important to spread protein intake throughout the day. Eating protein at key times—such as at breakfast, pre-workout, post-workout, and before bed—can support muscle repair, prevent muscle breakdown, and enhance performance. Whether your goal is to build muscle, maintain energy levels, or support your overall health, being mindful of when and how much protein you consume can have a significant impact on your progress.

Make Protein Your Best Friend

Protein isn't just for athletes or bodybuilders—it's a vital nutrient that supports every function in your body. From keeping your muscles strong to regulating your hormones, boosting your metabolism, and supporting your immune system, protein truly does it all.

The key to a healthy, sustainable diet is finding the right protein sources that fit your lifestyle. Whether you get it from animal-based foods, plant-based sources, or protein supplements, prioritizing protein will only benefit you in the long run.

So next time someone asks if you really need that extra serving of chicken, just remind them—you're fueling your body like a pro!

Fats – The Forgotten Heroes of Nutrition

When it comes to healthy eating, fats have been the villain in the story for way too long. For years, they were the poster child of all things bad for you — right alongside pizza after midnight and that extra glass of wine. The low-fat diet craze made us think fats were the enemy, the thing that would single-handedly ruin our health and our chances of fitting into skinny jeans. But hold up! In a plot twist that would make any soap opera jealous, science has done a full 180, and now we know fats are not only good for you but *essential* to your survival.

So, what gives? Why were fats public enemy number one for so long? Let's dive into the wonderful, misunderstood world of fats, and trust me, you'll soon be texting your avocado toast "thank you" messages.

What Are Fats?

Fats, also known as lipids (because, you know, it sounds fancier), are one of the three macronutrients — along with carbohydrates and proteins — that our body needs in bulk to keep us functioning like a well-oiled machine. While carbs are busy giving you a quick burst of energy, fats are the long-haulers. They're the reliable friend who sticks around for the marathon, not the sprint. For every gram of fat, you're getting 9 calories, which is more than double what you get from carbs or protein. So, while carbs might give you a short-term boost, fats are your ticket to *long-term energy* (think of them as your body's backup battery).

But fats aren't just here for the energy boost. They're also responsible for things like making hormones that regulate mood (so, if you're having a grumpy day, you know who to blame), metabolism, and growth. They form the very foundation of your cells—kind of like the brick and mortar of a house. And let's not forget, fats are the bodyguards of essential vitamins—A, D, E, and K—that keep your skin glowing, your bones strong, and your immune system firing on all cylinders. Oh, and they help protect your organs, too. Basically, fats are like the unsung superheroes of the body, but without the cape.

The Myths and Misunderstandings

Despite all these benefits, fats still have a bad reputation. One of the biggest myths is that all fats will lead to weight gain. Sure, fats are calorie-dense, but they also help keep you feeling full, so you're not raiding the fridge every five minutes like a snack-hungry zombie. Think of fats as your body's personal bouncer, preventing you from overdoing it on that extra bag of chips.

Another classic myth is that fats are bad for heart health. While there are some bad actors in the fat world (hello, trans fats and excessive saturated fats), there are plenty of good guys out there too. Healthy fats—like those found in avocados, nuts, and fatty fish—actually help protect your heart by reducing inflammation and improving cholesterol levels. So, the next time someone tells you that eating an avocado or egg yolk is a health crime, just smile and say, "I'm keeping my heart in check, thank you very much."

The truth about fats is simple: not all fats are created equal. The key is to focus on the healthy fats, and limit the unhealthy ones. When you get the balance right, fats aren't just safe—they're essential for your health. So, go ahead, grab that avocado toast (extra guac, please), and enjoy the benefits of fats as your body's trusted sidekick. After all, who knew the thing we once feared was the real MVP of our health journey?

The Different Types of Fats

Not all fats are created equal. Some are your body's bestie, while others are like that one friend who always cancels plans last minute. Understanding the different types of fats is crucial for making the best choices for your health, so let's break it down with a little humor, shall we?

Saturated Fats: The "Bad Boy" of the Fat World

Ah, the classic bad boy — *saturated fats*. These guys have been the villains in the health world for so long, they might as well have leather jackets and motorcycles. Saturated fats are solid at room temperature, which is why butter, cheese, and fatty meats are usually involved in any dramatic showdown. You'll also find them in tropical oils like coconut and palm oil (yes, those exotic oils we hear about when someone's trying to sell us a $30 jar of body lotion).

The thing is, saturated fats *do* raise cholesterol levels, but the whole "saturated fats = instant heart attack" narrative is a bit more complicated than we thought. Some studies suggest that not all saturated fats are heart-health villains. For instance, the saturated fats in coconut oil can raise HDL (that's the "good" cholesterol) and might even do some good. But if you're eating a steady diet of processed foods full of trans fats and sugar alongside your steak, then yeah, that's not exactly a recipe for good health.

The secret to navigating the saturated fat world? Moderation. Opt for quality sources like grass-fed beef, dairy from pasture-raised cows, and healthy tropical oils. But remember, a burger every now and then is fine, just don't turn it into a weekly affair.

Unsaturated Fats: The "Nice Guy" Fats

If saturated fats are the bad boys, unsaturated fats are like the sweet, reliable, always-gets-you-a-gift-for-your-birthday kind of person. These fats are liquid at room temperature, and they're often the "good fats" you hear about in all those *health food* blogs.

Trans Fats: The Fat That Should Be Banned From the Earth

And now, for the villain that even the worst *soap opera character* would be jealous of — *trans fats*. These guys are the worst because they're artificially created through a process called hydrogenation. That's right — someone actually *invented* these little monsters to make food last longer (because we all need a Twinkie that stays good for 100 years, right?).

Trans fats are found in many processed foods like margarine, packaged snacks, and fast food. They raise LDL (bad cholesterol) and lower HDL (good cholesterol), and basically make your heart run for the hills. The only good thing about trans fats is that most countries have stepped in and told them to *get lost*. So, to keep your heart happy and your arteries clear, just avoid trans fats altogether. Seriously, don't even *think* about them.

The Role of Fats in Your Body

Fats aren't just there to make you feel guilty about that extra slice of pizza — they're actually *really important* for your health! In fact, fats are like that reliable friend who's always there for you, even when you forget to call them. Let's dive into some of the key roles fats play in keeping your body running like a well-oiled machine (pun intended).

Energy Storage and Supply: The Backup Battery

Think of fat as your body's personal *backup battery* — like the one you keep in your drawer for when your phone's about to die, but way more important. When you eat more food than your body can immediately use, it stores the excess energy in fat cells, which act as your long-term fuel supply. During periods of fasting or intense physical activity (like that workout you said you'd do but haven't yet), the body taps into its fat reserves to keep you going. So yes, your fat is essentially your "get out of jail free" card when you're burning more energy than you're putting in.

Absorption of Fat-Soluble Vitamins: The VIP Pass

Fats are like the bouncers at the club, letting the VIP guests — vitamins A, D, E, and K — into the party. These fat-soluble vitamins are essential for your immune function, bone health, skin health, and even your vision. Without enough fat, your body can't properly absorb these critical nutrients, which is like throwing a party and not letting the good guests in. So, go ahead and embrace that drizzle of olive oil on your salad — your vitamins will thank you!

Cell Membrane Structure: The Body's Sticky Tape

Every single cell in your body has a membrane made of fat. Think of it as the body's version of sticky tape — keeping everything together and functioning smoothly. The fatty acids in these membranes allow nutrients and molecules to pass in and out, while maintaining the cell's structure like the best "security guard" on the block. Without fats, your cells would fall apart faster than a paper towel in a rainstorm.

Hormone Production: The Mastermind of Your Body's Drama

Let's talk hormones — those little messengers that run your life. Well, guess what? Fats, particularly cholesterol (the *good* kind, don't worry), are like the directors behind the scenes, producing hormones like estrogen, testosterone, and cortisol. These hormones manage everything from your metabolism to stress and even your mood. So next time you're feeling a little "hangry," just know that your fat is in there, helping to produce the right hormone to keep you from turning into a drama queen.

Brain Function: Your Brain's Favorite Snack

Did you know your brain is made up of about 60% fat? It's like the world's greatest avocado toast, but for your brain! Omega-3 fatty acids, in particular, are essential for keeping your brain sharp and functioning properly. They help form the structure of brain cells, support communication between neurons (those little brain messengers), and even improve mood and cognitive function. So, if you've ever wondered why you *can't remember where you left your keys,* just blame it on your lack of omega-3s, not your brain cells.

Protection of Organs and Temperature Regulation: The Body's Cushion

Think of fat as your body's personal bodyguard. Not only does it cushion your organs (just in case you have a little mishap while trying to impress someone with your dance moves), but it also acts as insulation to keep you warm in cold weather. So, if you've ever wondered why some people seem to be impervious to the cold, it's probably because their fat is doing its job and keeping them cozy. Maybe that extra layer of fluff is actually doing you a favor after all!

How Much Fat Do You Need?

Ah, fat. The macronutrient that's been vilified, praised, and then, somehow, praised again. But how much of it do you actually need? Let's break it down in a way that makes sense—and doesn't make you feel like you've just watched 10 YouTube videos on the Keto diet.

The Basics: Quantity Over Quality (But Not Too Much of Either)

The general rule of thumb is that 20-35% of your total daily calories should come from fat. That's enough to keep your body fueled and functioning like a well-oiled machine, without tipping the scales into "Why did I eat that entire pizza?" territory.

For example, if you're living the 2,000-calorie life (not too shabby), your daily fat intake should be between 44-78 grams. However, if you rely heavily on a high-carb diet, reducing your fat intake might be a smart choice.

Since both fats and carbs provide energy, it's essential to maintain a balanced ratio to avoid unnecessary weight gain. Often, fats get blamed, when in reality, an excess of carbs might be the real culprit.

Focus on Quality, Not Just Quantity (The Fat You Actually Want)

Not all fats are created equal, like how not all reality TV shows are *actually* "real" (looking at you, Kardashians). The quality of fat you consume is even more important than the quantity, because some fats are like that dependable friend who's always there for you, and others… well, they're more like that friend who borrows your stuff and never returns it.

Healthy fats, which are rich in monounsaturated and polyunsaturated fats, are your best friends. They improve heart health, reduce inflammation, and support brain function. They're like the "cool crowd" of the fat world. Some superstar sources of these fats include:

- Avocados: The Beyoncé of fats. Rich in monounsaturated fats, plus fiber, vitamins, and antioxidants. They're basically a party in your mouth and a health boost in your body.
- Nuts and Seeds (like almonds, walnuts, chia seeds, and flaxseeds): They're not just good for snacking; they're packed with monounsaturated fats, omega-3 fatty acids, and protein. Talk about multitasking.

- Olive Oil: The Mediterranean diet's secret weapon. It's like the smooth operator of healthy fats — full of anti-inflammatory compounds and heart-healthy monounsaturated fats.
- Fatty Fish (like salmon, mackerel, and sardines): These are the omega-3-rich superheroes your brain and heart adore. Omega-3s help your brain stay sharp (because who wants to forget where they put their keys again?).

On the flip side, some fats — like trans fats and excessive saturated fats — are more like the "bad boys" you should probably avoid. Trans fats, which hide in processed foods like baked goods, snacks, and margarine, raise bad cholesterol (LDL) while lowering good cholesterol (HDL), which sounds like a recipe for heart disease. Saturated fats (found in things like red meat and full-fat dairy) should be eaten in moderation. They're not as bad as we once thought, but they can still give your cholesterol levels a nasty surprise when consumed too much.

The Role of Fat in Your Diet: It's More Than Just Energy

Fat is more than just a fuel source. It's like the behind-the-scenes crew of a Broadway show — it does a lot of important stuff without asking for applause.

- Absorbing Vitamins: Fats help you absorb fat-soluble vitamins (A, D, E, and K). Without enough fat, your body can't properly absorb these vitamins, and your skin, bones, and vision might start to suffer. Imagine trying to enjoy a movie without the popcorn — just doesn't work, right?
- Cell Function: Every cell in your body is surrounded by a fat membrane, like a little fat fortress keeping everything intact. Without fat, your cells would fall apart like a badly planned Jenga tower.

- Hormone Production: Fat is also essential for hormone production. Without it, your hormone levels might go haywire, and we all know how much fun it is when that happens (note the sarcasm).
- Satisfaction: Fat helps you feel full longer, meaning you won't be raiding the kitchen every five minutes for a snack. It's like having a well-packed lunch box for your soul, keeping hunger at bay.

Be Mindful, Not Scared of Fat

Fat is calorie-dense — meaning you could eat a tiny bit and still rack up the calories pretty quickly. So, even though healthy fats are your friends, be mindful of portion sizes. It's easy to go overboard with nuts, seeds, and oils (guilty as charged with that avocado toast obsession).

The right amount of fat for you depends on your individual calorie needs, but aiming for 20-35% of your daily calories from fat is a solid start. Focus on healthy fats from sources like avocados, nuts, olive oil, and fatty fish, and try to limit trans fats and excessive saturated fats. This way, you can give your body the good fats it needs while avoiding the ones that make you regret that second helping of fries.

Embrace the Power of Fats

Fats have been the misunderstood, slightly neglected ingredient in the wellness world for far too long. They provide energy, support brain function, help regulate hormones, and even assist in absorbing those fancy fat-soluble vitamins (A, D, E, and K). So, instead of fearing fats, let's start showing them some love.

Opt for healthy fats — like those found in plant-based sources, fatty fish, and avocados — and try to keep the trans fats in check. With the right approach, fats can become the MVP of your diet. So go ahead, grab that avocado toast, toss some nuts in your salad, and embrace the wonderful world of healthy fats. You're doing your body a solid — and hey, you might even find yourself feeling a little more energized (and looking great doing it).

Water – The Elixir of Life (and Also Your Best Friend)

Water, the simple molecule made up of hydrogen and oxygen, is, without a doubt, the unsung hero of our bodies. It doesn't get the fame of coffee, the spotlight of pizza, or the everlasting popularity of chocolate, but it's arguably more essential to our survival than all of the above combined. Seriously, we could survive for weeks without food, but only a few days without water. If you think that's not impressive, you're wrong.

Water is like the oxygen of your diet – invisible, everywhere, and life-giving. While it doesn't make you feel like you're living your best life on its own (unless you're an overzealous water bottle enthusiast), it is, quite literally, keeping your body running like a finely-tuned machine. So, let's dive into the wonders of water, and why it should be the MVP of your daily routine.

What Is Water?

Water, my friend, is far more than just a beverage — it's the unsung hero of our existence. This simple compound, made up of two hydrogen atoms and one oxygen atom (H2O, for those who are still holding onto their high school chemistry knowledge), is responsible for so much more than just quenching your thirst. Water is the life force that keeps your body running smoothly, from maintaining proper hydration levels to flushing out toxins. Without it, you'd be an emotional mess, grumpy, sluggish, and — let's face it — miserable.

Water is crucial to almost every process in your body. Whether it's lubricating your joints, helping your body absorb nutrients, or aiding in digestion, water's role is indispensable. It also plays a huge part in regulating your body temperature, keeping you cool when you're sweating buckets on a hot day (or after an intense workout).

And let's not forget the ultimate multitasker: water helps to detoxify your body. It works tirelessly, like a cleanup crew, flushing out waste and ensuring your organs remain in tip-top shape. If you've ever wondered how your body stays healthy, look no further than the power of H2O. It's working day in and day out, maintaining balance and supporting overall health — sometimes without us even realizing it.

The Benefits of Water – Or Why Your Body Loves It

We all know the basic drill: water is essential for hydration. But let's dive a little deeper into what water actually does for your body. Spoiler alert: It's not just for quenching your thirst. Water is like that superhero we don't always acknowledge but couldn't live without. Whether you're running errands, working out, or even binge-watching your favorite show, water is silently working behind the scenes, keeping everything running smoothly. Here's why your body absolutely loves water:

1. Hydration – The Big One

Let's start with the obvious: hydration. Your body is made up of about 60% water. Yes, you read that right — your body is pretty much a walking water balloon. From your brain (which is about 75% water) to your muscles (about 79% water), and even your bones (which are about 31% water), water powers everything you do. It's the secret sauce that keeps your cells happy and functional. Imagine running a car engine without oil — your body's pretty much the same without adequate water. So, water is your engine oil, your high-octane fuel, and your coolant all rolled into one.

When you're well-hydrated, your body functions like a well-oiled machine.

2. Temperature Regulation – Your Built-in AC

Have you ever noticed how your body feels like it's giving up when you're dehydrated? Maybe your skin feels like it's been through the desert or you're too sluggish to move. That's because water plays a huge role in regulating your body temperature. When you sweat, you're losing water, but that's actually how your body keeps cool. The process of sweating allows your body to release heat, and guess what's in charge of all that? You guessed it—water. So, the next time you find yourself drenched in sweat after an intense workout (or, you know, walking to your car in the heat), remember that water is your built-in AC system, working hard to keep you cool.

3. Digestive Support – No More Cardboard Meals

Let's be real: We all love food, right? Whether it's a hearty meal or just some comfort snacks, we want our food to go down easy. But here's the thing: if you're not drinking enough water, your digestive system is basically just running in slow motion. Water helps break down food, ensuring your body can absorb nutrients efficiently. Without water, your digestion becomes sluggish, leaving you feeling bloated or uncomfortable. Imagine trying to eat cardboard—it's not exactly a smooth process, right? That's your body without enough water. So, next time you're indulging in your favorite foods, remember that water is the MVP making sure your body absorbs all the good stuff. Drink up, and your digestive system will thank you.

4. Detoxification – The Clean-Up Crew

Think of your body like a luxury apartment building. All sorts of toxins—like waste products and excess minerals—lurk around like that annoying neighbor who never does their laundry. But here's the twist: water is the maintenance worker who steps in to do a deep clean, sweeping up all the unwanted mess and leaving your body feeling fresh. It helps flush out waste, detoxify your system, and supports your kidneys in doing their job. Without enough water, your kidneys are like, "You serious? You're leaving us to clean this mess on our own?" And when your kidneys aren't working optimally, that's when you start feeling sluggish and tired. So, if you've been feeling off, water might just be the solution you've been missing.

5. Joint Lubrication – Smooth Moves Only

Remember how WD-40 keeps things moving smoothly when you're dealing with a squeaky door or stuck mechanism? Well, water is your body's version of WD-40. It helps lubricate your joints, keeping everything moving fluidly and pain-free. Whether you're running, walking, or even just bending down to pick something up, water is working to keep your joints from creaking like an old wooden floor. Without enough water, your joints can become stiff and sore, making it harder to move comfortably. So, the next time you feel like your body's starting to sound like a rusty car, remember—it's probably because you haven't been sipping enough H2O. Keep your joints oiled up with plenty of water, and you'll glide through life with ease.

How Much Water Do You Really Need?

We've all heard the classic "8 glasses a day" rule. But let's be real, sometimes that feels like a punishment, especially for those who aren't exactly water enthusiasts. Are you seriously going to chug that much water just because some health guru said so? Probably not. Here's the scoop: how much water you need really depends on your size, activity level, and climate. It's not a one-size-fits-all situation.

According to the Institute of Medicine, the average recommended daily intake is 3.7 liters (125 ounces) for men and 2.7 liters (91 ounces) for women. This includes water from food, beverages, and other liquids. So, yes, your cup of coffee or tea does count toward hydration. But, let's not get carried away and treat coffee as your main water source. After all, caffeine can act as a diuretic, making you pee more frequently, so it's probably best to balance it out with actual water.

Keep in mind that factors like exercise, weather, and even your diet (high-protein, high-sodium, or sugary foods can make you thirstier) can all impact how much water you need. If you're sweating buckets at the gym or it's a hot summer day, you might need more hydration. Listening to your body is key — if you're thirsty, drink.

Drinking Water – The Art of Sipping (or Gulping) Like a Pro

Drinking water may seem like a simple, straightforward task. But, let's be honest, it's not always as easy as it sounds. Sure, you could guzzle down a giant glass of water in one go and feel like you're winning at life, but if you want to give your body the best chance to absorb it and avoid running to the bathroom every 30 minutes, there's a better way: the art of sipping.

Here's how to turn your basic water-drinking routine into a fine-tuned hydration ritual:

1. Carry a Water Bottle Everywhere

Imagine you're at the beach, ready for a fun day in the sun. You wouldn't leave without sunscreen, right? Well, it's the same idea with a water bottle. Carry it with you everywhere – to work, the gym, the grocery store, or even just on a walk around the block. When you have it within arm's reach, sipping becomes second nature. The more you carry it, the less you forget to drink, and soon enough, staying hydrated will become as automatic as checking your phone. Plus, you'll look like you've got your life together, always ready to hydrate on the go. Bonus points for choosing a stylish bottle that matches your vibe.

2. Set Reminders

Let's be real: We all forget to drink water sometimes. Whether you're knee-deep in work, scrolling through TikTok, or binge-watching your latest obsession, hydration often takes a backseat. If you're guilty of that, don't worry – you're not alone. But here's the thing: setting reminders is a game-changer. Use your phone to set hourly alarms that remind you to take a sip. If you're feeling extra motivated, download one of those hydration apps that track your water intake and give you friendly (sometimes sassy) nudges to drink more. It's like having a little hydration coach in your pocket, except it doesn't judge you for procrastinating.

3. Spice It Up

Now, let's talk about flavor. If you find plain water a little too, well, plain, it's time to add some pizzazz! Water doesn't have to be boring. Try infusing it with fruits like lemon, lime, or berries, or add some cucumber or mint leaves for that spa-like vibe. Not only will your water look like it belongs in a fancy restaurant, but it will also taste like a million bucks. And let's be honest, anything that makes us feel a little fancier in our day-to-day lives is a win. You can even pretend you're sipping a mocktail at an upscale resort (minus the alcohol and the beach view). Pro tip: If you're feeling adventurous, throw in a few herbs or edible flowers for that extra touch of luxury.

4. Be a Water Snob

Alright, I'm not saying you have to be the person who only drinks water from a specific glacier or insists on artisanal bottled water (unless that's your thing, then more power to you). But it does help to find a water that you actually enjoy drinking. There's a whole world of water out there! Some people swear by sparkling water for that fizzy, refreshing feeling, while others prefer chilled spring water, feeling that it tastes fresher and cleaner. Explore your options! Find your "water soulmate," and suddenly, hydration won't feel like a chore. Whether it's water with a high mineral content or something as simple as filtered tap water, it's about discovering what works best for your taste buds.

5. *Savor Your Sips*

There's something to be said for taking your time with your water. Instead of gulping down large amounts in one go, take small, mindful sips throughout the day. You'll not only absorb it better, but you'll also give your body the steady hydration it needs. Plus, it's an opportunity to pause for a moment and enjoy a little break, whether you're in the middle of a hectic workday or just chilling on the couch. It's like giving yourself a mini refresh – one sip at a time.

6. *Hydration Goals*

Having a hydration goal can be just as satisfying as ticking off items from your to-do list. Set yourself a daily water target, whether it's aiming for that classic "8 glasses a day" or going for a higher goal based on your body's needs. It's a simple way to stay on track and make sure you're not neglecting your hydration. And when you hit your target? Feel free to give yourself a little celebratory fist bump. You've earned it.

7. *Switch Up Your Routine*

Sometimes, sticking to the same water routine day in and day out can feel like a drag. If you find yourself bored with your water, try changing things up. Alternate between regular water, flavored water, or sparkling water depending on your mood. You can also pair your hydration with healthy snacks like fruits or veggies, which contain water themselves, boosting your hydration game without you even realizing it. Remember: hydration doesn't just come from your water bottle – it's also in the foods you eat!

The Dangers of Dehydration – Why You Shouldn't Ignore Your Thirst

Dehydration is like that sneaky villain in a Bollywood thriller – it starts off quietly, maybe with just a few small signs that you can easily ignore. At first, you might feel a little sluggish, or perhaps, you notice a slight drop in your energy levels. Your skin might look a tad drier than usual, or you might find yourself getting cranky over the smallest things (hello, bad mood). But don't be fooled – this slow burn can quickly escalate into a much more serious problem if left unchecked.

In the sweltering heat of Indian summers, dehydration can sneak up on you faster than you'd think. Imagine walking around in the midday sun in Mumbai or Chennai – chances are you're sweating buckets, and all that sweat is your body's way of trying to cool itself down. But if you don't replenish that lost water, things can go south quickly. The symptoms can go from mild to severe: a dry mouth, dizziness, fatigue, and even a pounding headache. Your body can feel as though it's working overtime without any fuel.

But wait – things can get even worse. If dehydration continues unchecked, you might be in for more than just a headache. Chronic dehydration can lead to kidney stones (ouch!), urinary tract infections (UTIs), or even heat stroke. No one wants that, right? The thing is, dehydration is avoidable – if you listen to your body and stay ahead of it. When you feel thirsty, drink. When you feel irritable, drink. If you've been outside, sweating under the harsh sun, drink a lot of water. And we're talking *a lot*. Dehydration doesn't discriminate between morning joggers in Delhi or office workers in Bangalore; everyone is at risk if they ignore the signs.

It's a good rule of thumb to always have a water bottle with you. Keep a bottle in your bag, on your desk, or in your car. India's weather may be all over the place—from humid monsoon days in Kerala to hot desert air in Rajasthan—but your hydration needs stay constant. So, make water your best friend, especially during the hot months when dehydration is a serious risk.

The Myths About Water – Let's Set the Record Straight

India is a country rich in tradition, culture, and myths, and some of these myths have unfortunately found their way into our understanding of hydration. Let's clear up some of the most common water-related misconceptions so that you can drink smarter and stay healthier.

"You Must Drink 8 Glasses of Water a Day"

This one is the classic myth. We've all heard it: "8 glasses of water a day," and for many, this has become a non-negotiable rule. But the truth is, hydration needs vary from person to person. How much water you need depends on several factors—your body size, your activity level, the climate you live in, and even your diet. Someone living in the cooler hill stations of Himachal Pradesh might not need as much water as someone in the heat of Rajasthan. Plus, your food also contributes to your hydration needs. Fruits like watermelon and oranges and vegetables like cucumber are packed with water, so you're not just getting hydration from plain water. In short, drink enough to quench your thirst and keep your energy levels up. It's all about finding your own sweet spot, not sticking to a one-size-fits-all rule.

"Coffee and Tea Don't Count Towards Hydration"

Ah, the age-old debate—does tea or coffee count toward your daily water intake? The good news is, yes, it does! While it's true that caffeine is a diuretic (which means it can make you pee more), the amount of water in your coffee or chai still contributes to your overall hydration. In fact, Indians love their chai, and many of us drink it multiple times a day. So, don't let your morning cup of masala chai be your hydration villain. However, do keep in mind that excessive caffeine can have a dehydrating effect if you're drinking it in large amounts. So, while your morning cup of tea is a-ok, don't overdo the caffeine binge. After all, you're not trying to turn into a hyperactive squirrel running around all day.

"You Can't Drink Too Much Water"

Water is life, we all know that. But, surprise — *you can actually drink too much of it.* Drinking excessive amounts of water in a short period can dilute the electrolytes in your blood, leading to a condition known as hyponatremia (also known as water intoxication). This condition, though rare, can have serious consequences, including swelling of the brain, confusion, and in extreme cases, even death. So, while you might feel like a hydration superhero after downing two liters of water in an hour, it's essential to remember that moderation is key. Drinking small amounts of water throughout the day is much more effective than chugging a giant bottle all at once. So, don't get too carried away — your kidneys need time to process all that water.

"Water Doesn't Taste Like Anything, So It's Not Important"

Some people argue that water doesn't have a taste, so how important can it really be? Well, we're here to tell you that water is actually *the most important* part of your health. Sure, it might not have a fancy flavor like mango lassi or coconut water, but its role in maintaining body temperature, supporting digestion, flushing out toxins, and keeping your joints lubricated is undeniable. Water is the silent hero of your body, quietly doing all the heavy lifting behind the scenes.

"Drinking Water Only When You're Thirsty is Enough"

It's easy to assume that drinking when you're thirsty is all you need to do to stay hydrated. However, by the time you feel thirsty, your body may already be slightly dehydrated. Thirst is your body's way of saying, "Hey, I'm a little low on water here!" But at that point, you've probably already lost more water than you realize. So, make it a habit to drink water consistently throughout the day, even before you feel thirsty, especially if you're working in a hot climate or being physically active. Staying on top of hydration will help you avoid the dreaded effects of dehydration before they even start.

The bottom line is simple — water is essential to life, and you shouldn't ignore it. Dehydration can sneak up on you, so it's important to stay ahead of it by drinking regularly throughout the day. Water helps regulate your body temperature, flushes out toxins, aids in digestion, and keeps you feeling energized and focused.

Let's Raise a Glass (of Water)

Water, while it might not be as exciting as some other things we consume (like pizza or chocolate), is without a doubt the most important. It keeps everything functioning — your organs, your joints, and even your mood. So, next time you find yourself reaching for that third cup of coffee or gulping down sugary drinks, remember this: water is the original MVP.

The lesson here is simple: drink more water, stay hydrated, and embrace your newfound love for H2O. Your body will thank you — and you'll probably look a little less like a prune and a little more like someone who has their life together.

Now, go ahead. Grab that water bottle, sip it proudly, and know that you're one step closer to hydration greatness. Cheers!

Fibre – Your Gut's Best Friend (and Yours Too)

Fibre is like that quiet, underappreciated friend who always has your back but never gets enough credit. You know, the one who shows up at every party, ready to keep things running smoothly, but everyone's too busy admiring the loud, showy characters to notice. Well, let's give fibre its moment in the spotlight. Because, my friend, this nutrient is crucial to your well-being. It might not have the glamour of protein or the star power of carbs, but it deserves a standing ovation.

Fibre is an essential part of a healthy diet and plays a starring role in everything from digestion to heart health. And, contrary to popular belief, it's not just something you throw in your smoothie as an afterthought. No, no—it's time to take fibre seriously. And maybe have a laugh along the way, because fibre, like a good joke, works better when it's just right.

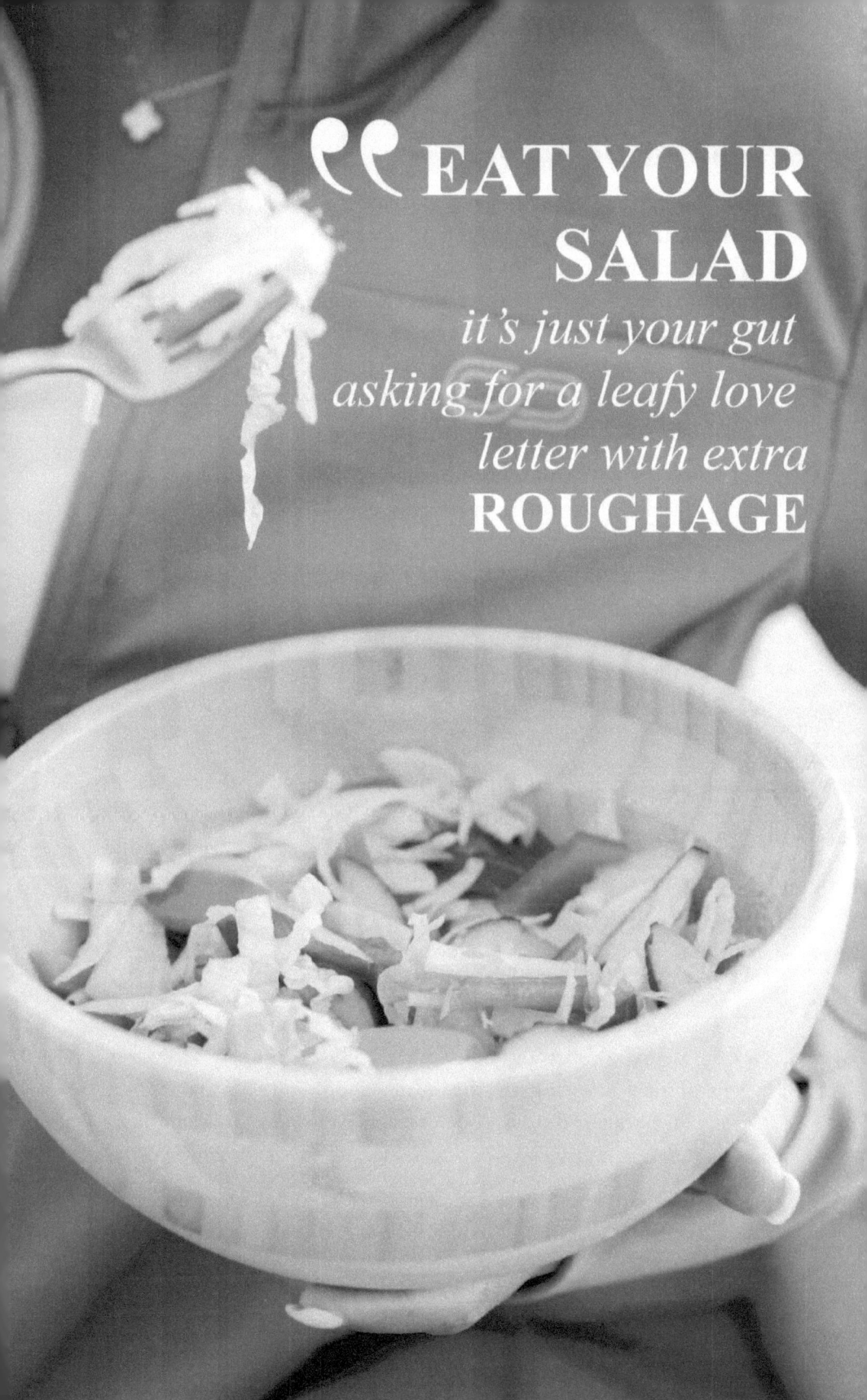

What is Fibre, Anyway?

First things first: what the heck is fibre? It's not some newfangled food trend or a superfood with a funny name. Fibre is actually a type of carbohydrate. But before you start imagining a carb-filled nightmare of pasta and bread, let's stop right there. Fibre isn't the kind of carbohydrate your body breaks down for energy. Instead, it's the part of plant-based foods that your body can't digest. Yes, you read that correctly — your body can't digest it. But that doesn't mean fibre isn't important. In fact, it's quite the opposite.

Fibre can be split into two types: soluble and insoluble. Soluble fibre dissolves in water and forms a gel-like substance in the stomach, helping to slow digestion and regulate blood sugar levels. Think of it as the "chill" fibre, helping you relax after a big meal. On the other hand, insoluble fibre doesn't dissolve in water. It helps to move food through your digestive system, preventing constipation and keeping things... well, moving. If soluble fibre is the chill one, insoluble fibre is the energetic, always-on-the-go sibling.

Both types of fibre are crucial to your health, but they work in different ways. Together, they form the dynamic duo that supports your digestive system like a dream team. But before we dive into all the amazing things fibre can do for you, let's talk about how much you actually need.

How Much Fibre Do You Really Need?

The answer is... it depends. There's no one-size-fits-all fibre recommendation because everyone's body is different. However, general guidelines suggest that adults should aim for about 25-30 grams of fibre per day. And before you panic and think you have to start eating entire fields of vegetables, let's break that down.

First, let's talk about how much fibre is in some common foods. One medium-sized apple has about 4 grams of fibre. A cup of cooked lentils packs around 15 grams. And don't forget about everyone's favorite "sneaky" source of fibre: whole grains. One slice of whole wheat bread can give you around 2 grams of fibre, so imagine how many slices you'd need to reach your daily goal (don't actually try that—your stomach might not appreciate it).

The trick to getting enough fibre is to gradually incorporate more of it into your meals, rather than trying to chug down an entire bag of bran in one sitting (please don't do that). If you slowly up your fibre intake, your body will thank you without revolting against you with bloating or discomfort.

The Digestive Superhero: Why Fibre is Important for Digestion

Now, let's get to the good stuff: why fibre is so important. The most obvious benefit is its role in digestion. As we mentioned earlier, fibre keeps things moving in your digestive system. It adds bulk to your stool, which helps to prevent constipation. If you've ever experienced that painful feeling of being backed up (and we're not talking about your email inbox), then you know how essential fibre is to a smooth, efficient digestive system.

Fibre is also fantastic at regulating your bowel movements. You've probably heard the phrase "regular as clockwork." Well, fibre is like your digestive system's personal assistant, making sure everything runs according to schedule. It absorbs water, swells up, and forms a soft, bulky stool that's easy to pass. No more straining and wondering why you feel like you're bench-pressing a weight every time you use the bathroom.

But it's not just about keeping things flowing; fibre also helps to maintain a healthy gut microbiome. Your gut is home to trillions of bacteria, and these bacteria are pretty important when it comes to digestion. Some types of fibre act as food for these good bacteria, helping them thrive. The better your gut bacteria are, the more efficient your digestion will be. So, in a way, fibre is like the VIP host at a party, ensuring that everyone has what they need to have a good time.

Fibre and Heart Health – A Love Story

Fibre doesn't just help you in the bathroom (though let's face it, that's a huge benefit). It's also fantastic for your heart. How, you ask? Well, research shows that a high-fibre diet is associated with a lower risk of heart disease. Soluble fibre, in particular, can help lower cholesterol levels. It binds to cholesterol in the digestive system and removes it from the body, preventing it from building up in your arteries.

In fact, if you're looking to lower your LDL cholesterol (the "bad" kind), fibre is a great place to start. You don't need to spend your life in a gym doing endless hours of cardio or pop cholesterol-lowering medications. Just add more fibre-rich foods to your diet, and you'll be doing your heart a huge favor.

So, next time you're munching on a bowl of oats or enjoying a handful of almonds, know that you're doing more than just satisfying your taste buds — you're also taking care of your heart. It's like getting a free pass to eat snacks that are good for you. Who knew health could taste so good?

Fibre and Weight Management – Your New Best Friend

If you're trying to maintain a healthy weight (or even lose a few kilos), fibre can be your ally. Fibre-rich foods take longer to chew and digest, which means you'll feel fuller for longer. This helps to curb unnecessary snacking and overeating. So, the next time you're tempted to grab a packet of chips, try reaching for some veggies, fruits, or a handful of seeds instead. They'll keep you satisfied and help you avoid those mid-afternoon snack cravings.

But it's not just about making you feel full — it's also about how fibre interacts with your digestive system. High-fibre foods tend to be lower in calories, meaning you can eat larger portions without consuming an excess of calories. Plus, fibre slows down the absorption of sugar, helping to regulate blood sugar levels. So, no more blood sugar spikes and crashes that leave you feeling like you've just run a marathon.

In short, fibre helps you maintain a balanced diet, feel satisfied with your meals, and regulate your blood sugar — all key factors when it comes to managing weight.

Fibre-Rich Foods to Add to Your Diet

Now that we've established that fibre is a true hero for your gut and overall health, let's take a deeper dive into the foods that can provide you with all the fibre goodness you need. These foods will not only help you stay regular but also support your heart health, manage weight, and keep your digestive system in top shape. Ready for the fibre-filled ride? Let's go!

1. Fruits: Nature's Fibre Powerhouses

Fruits are like nature's candy — but with a lot more benefits. They're sweet, satisfying, and packed with fibre that helps keep your digestive system running smoothly. Some of the best options include:

- Apples: A medium-sized apple contains about 4 grams of fibre, mostly from the skin. Apples are not only crunchy and delicious but also easy to carry as a snack.

- Pears: A pear is another fibre-packed fruit. One medium-sized pear can provide up to 5-6 grams of fibre. It's juicy, refreshing, and perfect for satisfying your sweet cravings.

- Berries: Strawberries, blueberries, raspberries, and blackberries are all fibre-rich fruits. A cup of raspberries, for example, can deliver a whopping 8 grams of fibre! Add them to smoothies, yogurts, or just eat them as a snack.

- Bananas: While bananas are often known for their potassium content, they also have a decent amount of fibre, especially when slightly green. Bananas make for a quick, satisfying snack with about 3 grams of fibre per medium banana.
- Oranges: Full of vitamin C, oranges are also a good source of soluble fibre. One medium orange provides about 3-4 grams of fibre and a sweet burst of hydration.

2. Vegetables: Fibre from the Green Team

Vegetables aren't just good for your body; they're also great for your gut. High in fibre, these plant foods help keep your digestive system in tip-top shape. Some top contenders include:

- Broccoli: Known for its cancer-fighting properties, broccoli also packs a decent amount of fibre. One cup of cooked broccoli contains around 5 grams of fibre, making it a great addition to soups, stir-fries, and salads.
- Brussels Sprouts: These little cabbages are packed with both soluble and insoluble fibre. One cup of Brussels sprouts contains 4 grams of fibre. Roasted or steamed, they make a tasty side dish.
- Carrots: Crunchy, sweet, and high in fibre, carrots are a great snack option. One medium carrot has about 2 grams of fibre. Toss them into salads or munch on them raw with hummus for a fibre boost.
- Spinach: Spinach is a low-calorie vegetable that's loaded with fibre. A cup of cooked spinach contains about 4 grams of fibre. You can add it to your smoothies, curries, or as a side dish.
- Sweet Potatoes: Not only are sweet potatoes delicious, but they're also a fibre powerhouse. A medium-sized sweet

potato has about 4 grams of fibre, particularly in the skin. Try them roasted, mashed, or as fries for a fibre-packed treat.

3. Legumes: The Fibre Rich Superfoods

Legumes are often overlooked, but they are incredible sources of both soluble and insoluble fibre. These plant-based proteins are excellent for your digestive system and overall health. Some great legumes to include are:

- Lentils: A fantastic source of fibre and protein, lentils provide about 15 grams of fibre per cooked cup. Add them to soups, stews, or salads, or make a lentil curry for a filling, fibre-rich meal.
- Chickpeas: Also known as garbanzo beans, chickpeas are a versatile legume. One cup of cooked chickpeas has about 12 grams of fibre. Use them in hummus, salads, or curries for a delicious and satisfying meal.
- Black Beans: Black beans are another excellent source of fibre. A cup of cooked black beans delivers around 15 grams of fibre. Toss them into tacos, burritos, or make a hearty bean soup.
- Kidney Beans: Kidney beans, with their rich red color, are high in fibre and protein. One cup of cooked kidney beans contains about 13 grams of fibre. Add them to stews, salads, or chili for a hearty, fibre-filled meal.

4. Whole Grains: Carb-Lovers, Rejoice

Whole grains are often misunderstood, with many people fearing carbs. But when it comes to whole grains, they're actually a fibre-filled friend. These grains provide steady energy while keeping your digestive system happy. Some top picks are:

- Oats: Oats are a great source of soluble fibre, specifically beta-glucan, which can help lower cholesterol. A cup of cooked oats has about 4 grams of fibre. Enjoy them as oatmeal, in smoothies, or in baked goods.

- Quinoa: A protein-rich grain that also delivers a healthy dose of fibre, quinoa provides about 5 grams of fibre per cooked cup. It's perfect as a base for salads, bowls, or as a side dish.
- Millets: Millets are a powerhouse of fiber, aiding digestion, regulating blood sugar, and promoting gut health. These ancient grains keep you full longer, support weight management, and provide sustained energy throughout the day.

5. Nuts and Seeds: The Snackable Fibre Boosters

Nuts and seeds are not just for making nut butter or sprinkling on granola. They're rich in fibre and healthy fats that will keep you feeling satisfied. Here are a few fibre-rich snacks to consider:

- Almonds: Almonds are a great source of both soluble and insoluble fibre. A handful (about 23 almonds) contains around 3.5 grams of fibre. Snack on them, add them to salads, or mix them into your morning yogurt.
- Chia Seeds: Chia seeds are tiny but mighty when it comes to fibre. Just two tablespoons of chia seeds provide about 10 grams of fibre. Add them to smoothies, overnight oats, or even make chia pudding for a nutritious treat.
- Flaxseeds: Flaxseeds are another fibre-packed powerhouse. Two tablespoons of ground flaxseeds deliver around 4 grams of fibre. Sprinkle them on cereal, blend them into smoothies, or use them as an egg replacement in baking.

Fibre, The Unsung Hero

Fibre may not be the most glamorous nutrient in the food world, but it's certainly one of the most important. From keeping your digestive system running smoothly to supporting heart health, weight management, and even your gut microbiome, fibre is truly a jack-of-all-trades.

So, the next time you bite into that juicy apple or enjoy a hearty bowl of dal, remember that you're not just feeding your body — you're nourishing it. Fibre may not always steal the spotlight, but it's definitely the backstage crew making sure everything goes off without a hitch.

Incorporate more fibre into your diet, and your body will thank you. You'll be feeling healthier, more energetic, and more regular than ever before. And let's face it, who wouldn't want that?

Beverages: The Liquid Side of Life

Think about it — beverages have always been there, quietly anchoring our days. Before we even think of food, most of us instinctively reach for a drink. A glass of water, a hot cup of chai, a protein shake, lemon water with turmeric — each choice says something about who we are and how we're feeling in that moment.

Because we don't just drink to hydrate.

We drink to *feel*.

Sometimes it's ritual — a warm mug clasped between sleepy fingers before the world begins to stir. Other times, it's routine. A mid-morning soda, an iced latte just before lunch, a kombucha at sundown because, well, your gut deserves it. We drink to energize, to unwind, to soothe, to celebrate. And sometimes, we drink just to have something to hold.

Beverages carry emotion. They're offered before questions, shared during heartbreak, gossip, celebration, and change.

They tell stories — of culture, of habits, of us.

From a cold glass of chaas in the Indian summer, to ceremonial matcha in Japan, to green juice in a post-yoga LA glow — every sip holds more than ingredients. It holds intention.

And when it comes to daily brews, two reign supreme: ***tea and coffee.***

Why are we focusing on tea and coffee here? Because these two beloved beverages, though deeply embedded in our daily routines, are often consumed in ways that do more harm than good. Most people reach for their morning cup of tea or coffee as a ritual—something to wake them up, get their day started, or simply offer comfort. But what's rarely considered is how we're consuming them, when, and in what form.

Consuming tea or coffee first thing in the morning, especially on an empty stomach, can disrupt cortisol levels, spike acidity, and even lead to hormonal imbalances over time. The combination of caffeine with sugar, processed creamers, or milk can burden the digestive system and, in some cases, exacerbate bloating, fatigue, or skin issues. What starts as a simple morning habit can slowly chip away at your gut health and energy levels without you even realizing it.

That's why it's essential to re-evaluate these daily beverages—not to cut them out completely, but to understand their impact and consume them in a way that supports your well-being.

Tea, with its roots steeped in ceremony and calm, is often seen as the gentler choice—soothing, grounding, thoughtful. From herbal blends to spicy chais, it's a drink of healing and reflection.

Coffee, on the other hand, is bold and awakening. It's the brew of ambition, powering deadlines, morning commutes, and creative bursts. It sharpens, uplifts, and commands attention with every strong sip.

So—what's in your cup?

Are you a coffee person, or does tea rule your world? As a nutritionist, I constantly get asked, *"Are teas or coffees good for you?" "Which one's better?" "Do they have any nutritional value?" "When and how should we consume them?"* Well, let's dive in and uncover the truth behind your favorite drinks.

<u>The real culprit? It's not caffeine. It's the milk and sugar we dump into them mindlessly</u>. So before you blame your cup of coffee or tea, ask yourself: *Is it really about the caffeine, or do you just crave that hit of sweetness and dairy in the morning?*

Coffee: The Good, The Bad, and The Bitter Truth

You know the feeling. You've barely opened your eyes, and your hand's already reaching for the coffee machine. That first whiff? Instant comfort. That first sip? Life officially begins.

For most of us, coffee isn't just a beverage—it's a ritual we don't dare skip. It powers our 9 AM meetings, fuels our deadlines, and sometimes just gets us through conversations we didn't sign up for. Whether it's the local café knowing your "usual" or the silent nod you give your mug every morning, there's a familiarity in coffee that feels oddly intimate. It wakes us up, sets the tone, and for a lot of us—it feels like control in a chaotic world.

And for fitness lovers? Coffee becomes a pre-workout kick, a quick-fix energy booster to hit that extra rep or run that final mile. It's all part of the hustle.

But here's the thing—we rarely stop to ask *why* we need it so much. Or what that third cup might be doing to our gut, hormones, or sleep. Is coffee our friend, or a frenemy in disguise?

Let's dive deeper into what this beloved brew really does to your body—from the highs and the hidden harms, to the dos and don'ts that could make all the difference.

The Facts:

- **Caffeine spikes cortisol:** Drinking coffee first thing in the morning, especially on an empty stomach, can cause a surge in cortisol (your stress hormone). This can lead to increased anxiety, disrupted blood sugar levels, and hormonal imbalances over time.

- **It's a diuretic:** Coffee can dehydrate you, especially if you're not balancing it with enough water. This dehydration can impact digestion, skin health, and energy levels.
- **It can mess with your gut:** Coffee stimulates acid production, which can irritate the stomach lining—leading to bloating, acid reflux, or even gut inflammation for some people.
- **It disrupts sleep:** Caffeine has a half-life of about 5-6 hours, which means that late-afternoon cup could be quietly sabotaging your sleep quality—even if you *think* it's not.

Dos:

- **Do** wait 60-90 minutes after waking up before your first cup to allow natural cortisol levels to balance.
- **Do** hydrate first—start your day with water (bonus: add lemon or electrolytes) before reaching for caffeine.
- **Do** pair coffee with a meal or healthy fat (like coconut oil or ghee) to reduce its harsh impact on your stomach lining.
- **Do** opt for organic, mold-free coffee when possible, especially if you're sensitive to gut issues or inflammation.
- **Do** try herbal or adaptogenic alternatives occasionally (like chicory root or ashwagandha blends) to give your body a break.

Don'ts:

- **Don't** rely on coffee as a meal replacement—this spikes cortisol and drops blood sugar, leading to cravings and energy crashes.
- **Don't** have coffee on an empty stomach, especially if you're already dealing with gut issues, PCOS, or thyroid imbalances.
- **Don't** consume caffeine after 2-3 PM if you're sensitive to sleep disruptions.

- **Don't** overdo it — more isn't better. 1-2 cups of coffee can be beneficial, but 4-5 might be working against you.

Why Not Coffee First Thing in the Morning?

You've been fasting for 8-10 hours while you sleep. Your body wakes up in a dehydrated state, and the first thing you feed it? A diuretic that flushes out even more water. Yep, that's coffee for you. Drinking coffee on an empty stomach can:

- Spike cortisol levels, which can lead to increased stress and anxiety.
- Cause digestive issues, as caffeine stimulates acid production and may irritate the stomach lining.
- Lead to dehydration, making you feel sluggish instead of energized.

So what should you do instead? Start your day with electrolytes and water, then go for something gentler like ginger turmeric tea before indulging in caffeine.

The Benefits of Coffee

But don't get me wrong — I love coffee! It's that little ritual that fuels my day and gets me going. When consumed mindfully, coffee has several health benefits that go beyond just waking you up:

- **Heart Health** - Coffee is packed with antioxidants, which help protect your heart by fighting off harmful inflammation. It's like giving your heart a little protective shield with every sip.
- **Brain Function** - You've probably felt it firsthand: that mental clarity after your first cup. Coffee helps improve focus, lift your mood, and keep your brain sharp — making it the perfect go-to when you need to tackle tasks or power through your to-do list.

- **Metabolism Booster** – If you've ever felt that buzz from coffee, it's not just in your head. Caffeine helps rev up your metabolism, speeding up fat oxidation and increasing energy production. So yeah, your body's burning a bit more fuel just by sipping that cup.
- **Digestive Support** – For some, coffee works as a gentle kick to the digestive system, helping things move along like clockwork. For others, though, it can be a little harsh. It all comes down to your gut bacteria, which determines whether coffee will give you that helpful push — or leave you feeling a bit bloated.
- **Pre-Workout** – That little jolt you get from your morning cup? It's not just for getting you through the day. Coffee's caffeine is great for boosting energy and performance during workouts, giving you that extra endurance when you hit the gym or go for a run. It's like a pre-workout, but way more affordable!

When and How Much Coffee Should You Have?

The golden rule? 1-2 cups per day is ideal. Avoid drinking it:

- First thing in the morning (wait at least 60-90 minutes after waking up)
- On an empty stomach (always pair it with food if your gut is sensitive)
- Too late in the day (caffeine has a half-life of 5-6 hours, meaning it lingers in your system and can disrupt sleep)

The Coffee Spectrum: Light vs. Medium vs. Dark Roast

Coffee lovers know that not all brews are created equal — your choice of roast can completely transform the flavor, caffeine kick, and overall experience of your cup. From the bright and fruity light roast to the bold and smoky dark roast, each has its own charm.

Light roast coffee is the golden child for those who love a bright, acidic, and slightly fruity flavor. Because it's roasted for the shortest amount of time, it retains the most caffeine, making it the perfect choice for an early morning energy boost. If you enjoy the delicate complexities of coffee, a light roast will let you savor its natural flavors without the deeper, caramelized notes that come with longer roasting.

Medium roast strikes the perfect balance—smooth, nutty, and slightly caramelized, it's the go-to choice for everyday coffee drinkers. It offers a moderate caffeine content and a well-rounded taste that's neither too acidic nor too bitter. If you're looking for a crowd-pleaser that can be enjoyed black or with milk, medium roast is your best bet.

For those who prefer a bold, full-bodied cup, dark roast is the way to go. With its smoky, slightly bitter profile, this roast has a rich depth that espresso lovers adore. Despite its intense flavor, dark roast actually contains the least amount of caffeine due to the longer roasting process breaking down more of the coffee's natural stimulant. It also has lower acidity, making it a great option for those with sensitive stomachs.

Whether you need a bright and zesty wake-up call, a smooth and balanced daily brew, or a bold and comforting sip, the roast you choose sets the stage for your coffee experience. So, what's in your cup today?

Why I Prefer Light Roast

Personally, I love light roast coffee because it preserves the bean's original flavors—citrusy, floral, and vibrant. Plus, it has the highest caffeine content, making it a great morning pick-me-up. Dark roast, on the other hand, loses a lot of its natural notes and tends to taste burnt, which doesn't appeal to me.

***

While coffee is a beloved staple for many, sometimes you might crave a gentler, more health-focused alternative. Enter **green coffee**—a lesser-known version of your favorite brew that's gaining popularity for its subtle benefits. If you've ever wondered if there's a way to enjoy the perks of coffee without the jitters or the intensity, green coffee might just be the answer you've been looking for.

Green Coffee: The Unroasted Super Brew

You've probably heard the buzz around green coffee recently and wondered what all the hype is about. If you're used to your regular cup of joe, you might be thinking, "Why would I switch?" Well, green coffee isn't just some trend—it's a healthier, gentler alternative that packs a punch with its benefits.

Unlike your typical brew, which is made from roasted beans, green coffee is made from unroasted ones, leaving all those natural compounds intact. One of its star players is chlorogenic acid, a powerful antioxidant known for its role in regulating blood sugar and supporting fat metabolism. So, if you've been looking for a way to balance your energy and metabolism without the crash or jitters of regular coffee, green coffee could be your answer.

Now, let's talk about the flavor. Green coffee is a little more subtle, with a mild, herbal taste that's a nice change from the bold, often bitter notes of regular coffee. It's caffeine, but with a softer, steadier kick—perfect for those days when you need a boost but don't want to feel overstimulated.

But the benefits don't stop there. Studies show that green coffee can also support heart health by reducing inflammation and promoting healthy blood pressure levels. It's like a calming, nurturing sip for both your body and mind.

If you're ready to break from your usual routine or just want to try something that's both comforting and nourishing, green coffee might be exactly what you need. Whether you brew it like tea, sip it as an extract, or enjoy it as a daily habit, it's a refreshing way to get your caffeine fix without the added heaviness of traditional coffee. So, why not give it a try and see if green coffee becomes your new favorite brew?

***

When someone says "green drink," your mind might immediately jump to kale smoothies or even your morning coffee in a green tumbler. But there's a new star steeping in the spotlight—and no, it's not just a trend. It's matcha.

Once a quiet staple in Japanese tea ceremonies, matcha has now taken center stage in our global wellness rituals. It's earthy, smooth, and carries a kind of gentle focus that no other caffeine can quite match. No jitters. No crash. Just calm energy and clarity in every sip.

From cozy corners of your favorite indie cafés to the sleek kitchen counters of influencers who somehow glow from within, matcha is everywhere. Whisked into creamy lattes, baked into cookies, blended into smoothies—matcha isn't just a drink anymore; it's a lifestyle choice. A soft flex. A green badge of wellness.

Why the obsession? Maybe it's the antioxidants. Maybe it's the ritual of whisking and pouring. Or maybe, it's the way matcha makes you feel: like you're treating yourself and taking care of yourself at the same time.

Matcha: The Zen Superfood in a Cup

So, you've probably heard of matcha by now, right? It's not just another trendy drink—it's a powerhouse of energy, focus, and antioxidants. Rooted deeply in Japanese tradition, matcha isn't your typical tea. While regular green tea is steeped and discarded, matcha uses the whole leaf, finely ground into a powder, so you're consuming all the nutrients. This makes it significantly richer in antioxidants, especially catechins, which help fight oxidative stress and support overall health.

One of the best things about matcha is how it gives you a steady, sustained energy boost without that dreaded caffeine crash. Unlike coffee, matcha contains caffeine, but it also has an amino acid called L-theanine that calms the mind and enhances focus. This unique combination results in a smooth, jitter-free energy release, making matcha the go-to for people who need to stay sharp and focused — whether for work, study, or even meditation.

But matcha isn't just about keeping you awake. It has plenty of other health benefits. It helps with metabolism and fat oxidation, making it a favorite for those focusing on weight management. It's also packed with chlorophyll, which helps detox the body by removing toxins and heavy metals. Plus, matcha has been linked to improved heart health by lowering bad cholesterol and regulating blood pressure.

And let's talk about preparation — it's an experience in itself. Traditionally, matcha is whisked into hot water to create a frothy, vibrant green drink. But if you're into modern twists, matcha lattes, smoothies, and even baked goods are becoming popular options. Whether you drink it for focus, energy, or health, matcha is more than a trend — it's a lifestyle choice that's worth sipping.

***

Tea – A World of Wellness in a Cup

There's something sacred about that first sip of chai. The steam curling up from the cup, the familiar scent of ginger, cardamom, and cloves wrapping around you like a hug — it's more than just a drink. It's a ritual. A mood-setter. A cultural comfort that says, *"Take a breath. You're home."*

For many of us, chai is how the day begins, how breaks are punctuated, and how conversations deepen. It's in the shared moments with family, the pause between chaos, the quiet after a storm. It's warm, nostalgic, and deeply rooted in our routines.

But sometimes, those rituals can quietly shift into habits that don't serve us as well anymore.

Too much sugar. Too much milk. Three cups before noon. Four by bedtime. Caffeine dependence sneaking in disguised as comfort. And slowly, what once grounded us starts to leave us feeling drained, jittery, or bloated. That's where the reset comes in — not by abandoning the ritual, but by reimagining it.

Enter: Healing Teas. These aren't just trendy tisanes with pretty names. They're functional, intentional, and deeply restorative. Think tulsi when your stress levels spike. Chamomile when your sleep's been off. Peppermint to ease digestion. Ashwagandha to anchor your nervous system. Or fennel and ajwain when your gut's throwing tantrums.

Replacing that third chai of the day with a healing tea doesn't mean giving up comfort — it means choosing comfort that gives back. It's still about the warmth in your hands, the breath you take as you sip, the pause in your day. But now, that moment is infused with purpose.

So maybe we don't need to quit chai — we just need to redefine our rituals. Bring back the intention. Bring back the care. Let your cup hold healing.

Caffeinated Teas – The Natural Pick-Me-Up

For those looking for a balanced source of energy, caffeinated teas offer the perfect solution. Unlike coffee, which delivers a rapid caffeine spike, tea provides a more sustained energy release, thanks to the presence of L-theanine, an amino acid that promotes calm alertness. With a variety of flavors, caffeine levels, and health benefits, there's a tea for every moment of the day. Let's explore some] of the most popular caffeinated teas and what makes them stand out.

Black Tea – The Bold Classic

Black tea is the strongest of all traditional teas, both in terms of flavor and caffeine content. With its rich, malty taste, black tea is a great alternative to coffee for those who enjoy a strong, full-bodied brew. It contains a high level of caffeine, making it the perfect morning or afternoon drink for an instant pick-me-up.

Beyond its energizing properties, black tea is packed with antioxidants called flavonoids, which support heart health by improving circulation and reducing inflammation. Additionally, it enhances cognitive function, sharpening focus and mental clarity. Whether enjoyed plain or with milk and sugar, black tea is a timeless favorite for those seeking both energy and wellness.

Earl Grey – The Elegant Mood Booster

A variation of black tea, Earl Grey stands out due to its infusion of bergamot oil, which gives it a distinctive citrusy and floral aroma. This tea is not only refreshing but also a great mood enhancer. The combination of caffeine and the soothing scent of bergamot makes it an excellent choice for mid-morning or afternoon consumption.

Earl Grey is known to help alleviate stress and anxiety, thanks to the calming properties of bergamot. It also aids digestion, making it a great option after meals. If you're looking for a tea that offers both a mental boost and relaxation in a single cup, Earl Grey is a sophisticated choice.

Oolong Tea – The Metabolism Booster

Oolong tea is the perfect middle ground between black and green tea, offering a smooth, floral taste with a moderate caffeine level. What sets oolong apart is its metabolism-boosting benefits. Rich in polyphenols, this tea helps regulate fat metabolism, making it an excellent choice for those looking to support weight management.

Additionally, oolong tea is beneficial for gut health. It promotes digestion and maintains a healthy balance of gut bacteria, reducing bloating and digestive discomfort. The best time to drink oolong is before meals, as it prepares the digestive system for optimal nutrient absorption.

Green Tea – The Antioxidant Powerhouse

Green tea is widely celebrated for its health benefits. With a fresh, slightly bitter taste, it contains a moderate amount of caffeine, making it a great alternative for those who want an energy boost without over-stimulation. It's particularly effective before workouts, as it enhances fat oxidation and provides a steady flow of energy.

Loaded with catechins, green tea is an antioxidant powerhouse that fights oxidative stress and supports overall well-being. It's also known for improving brain function, boosting metabolism, and reducing the risk of chronic diseases. Whether enjoyed plain or as a matcha latte, green tea is a smart choice for health-conscious individuals.

Non-Caffeinated Teas – Healing & Relaxation

For those seeking warmth, comfort, and wellness without the stimulating effects of caffeine, non-caffeinated teas offer a soothing alternative. These herbal infusions are packed with antioxidants, vitamins, and healing properties that support digestion, relaxation, and overall well-being. Whether you're winding down for bed, easing digestive discomfort, or boosting immunity, there's a non-caffeinated tea to suit every need.

Peppermint Tea – The Digestive Soother

With its cool, refreshing taste, peppermint tea is a go-to remedy for digestive issues. It helps relax the digestive tract, reducing bloating, gas, and indigestion. Its natural menthol content provides a cooling sensation that soothes the stomach and promotes overall gut health. Peppermint tea is best enjoyed after meals to aid digestion and provide a refreshing burst of flavor.

Blue Pea Tea – The Brain-Boosting Beauty Elixir

Also known as butterfly pea flower tea, this striking blue infusion is rich in antioxidants that support brain health, enhance memory, and promote glowing skin. Its mild, earthy, and floral taste makes it a gentle, calming drink that can be enjoyed at any time of the day. When mixed with lemon, the tea changes color from blue to purple, making it not only a healthful choice but also a visually stunning one.

Hibiscus Tea – The Heart's Best Friend

With a tart, fruity flavor reminiscent of cranberries, hibiscus tea is known for its ability to lower blood pressure and support heart health. It's packed with vitamin C, which boosts immunity and fights inflammation. Hibiscus tea is perfect for an afternoon refreshment, offering a cooling effect that makes it a great iced tea option as well.

Lavender Tea – The Stress Reliever

Lavender tea is a floral, mild infusion known for its ability to calm the mind and ease anxiety. Its soothing properties make it an excellent choice for unwinding after a long day. Drinking lavender tea in the evening helps promote relaxation and prepares the body for restful sleep. It's also beneficial for headaches and stress relief, making it a wonderful self-care ritual.

Chamomile Tea – The Sleep Enhancer

Chamomile tea is often associated with bedtime due to its calming effects. With a naturally sweet, apple-like flavor, it relaxes the nervous system, reduces stress, and aids digestion. Chamomile tea is particularly beneficial for those who struggle with insomnia, making it the perfect nightcap to ensure a peaceful sleep.

Kahwa (Kashmiri Tea) – The Warming Immunity Booster

A traditional Kashmiri tea, kahwa is an aromatic blend of green tea, saffron, cardamom, and almonds, offering a rich, spiced flavor. Though it's caffeine-free, it provides warmth and energy, making it ideal for cold mornings. Packed with antioxidants, kahwa supports immunity, improves digestion, and keeps the body warm during winter.

Cinnamon Tea – The Metabolism Regulator

With its warm, spicy flavor, cinnamon tea is a powerful anti-inflammatory and blood sugar regulator. It aids in digestion, boosts metabolism, and helps control sugar cravings. The best time to drink cinnamon tea is in the morning or before meals to stabilize blood sugar levels and support weight management.

Ginger Turmeric Tea – The Anti-Inflammatory Powerhouse

A blend of ginger and turmeric creates a potent tea with strong anti-inflammatory properties. This earthy, spicy infusion is excellent for gut health, reducing inflammation, and boosting immunity. Drinking it first thing in the morning helps kickstart digestion and provides a natural detox for the body.

***

A Warm Embrace in Every Sip

Warm beverages are more than just drinks — they are a source of comfort, healing, and nourishment. They support our detox system, aid digestion, and provide moments of relaxation in our fast-paced lives. Personally, I'm a fan of light roast coffee because it's the freshest, most vibrant way to enjoy coffee. Roasted at lower temperatures (350-400°F), it retains more of its natural flavors and has the highest caffeine content — making it my go-to for an energizing start to the day. Its bright acidity and fruity, citrusy notes make each sip feel light and refreshing. In contrast, dark roast coffee, with its smoky, bitter, and burnt taste, doesn't appeal to me. It loses much of the bean's original flavor and contains less caffeine, which doesn't align with my energy needs.

However, as much as I love coffee, I don't believe in consuming caffeine first thing in the morning. It dehydrates the body and spikes cortisol levels unnecessarily. That's why I always start my day with electrolytes to hydrate myself, followed by a ritual of ginger turmeric tea. This tea is a powerhouse for reducing inflammation, improving gut health, and preventing bloating — making it one of the most important teas for overall well-being.

In the evening, I switch to chamomile tea, known for its calming properties and ability to promote restful sleep. Not just for me, but I also recommend this ritual to my clients who often overindulge in caffeine. It's about finding balance — choosing the right caffeine source that works for you while avoiding unnecessary additives like milk and sugar. That way, you can truly experience the real, rich flavors of your beverage without the need for anything sweet or creamy.

WHICH DIET?
OH! SUCH A DILEMMA!

Mediterranean Diet
Keto Diet
Paleo Diet
Vegan Diet
DASH Diet
Calorie Deficit
Whole-30 Diet
Low Carb Diet
Intermittent Fasting

Diet Dilemmas: The Battle of the Diets (And Which One Might Actually Work for You)

In a world where every other influencer has a "secret diet" that promises to change your life, it's easy to get lost in the whirlwind of health trends. One moment you're debating between avocado toast or kale chips, and the next, someone's telling you that fasting for 16 hours is the key to unlocking your ultimate self. With so many options — Mediterranean, Keto, Whole30, and the occasional new "miracle diet" popping up every week — how do you make sense of it all without going crazy (or hungry)? Well, don't worry. We're here to navigate this maze of meals, break down the pros and cons of each diet, and hopefully add some humor to this food-for-thought journey. Because, let's face it, life's too short to take every diet trend too seriously — especially when there's pizza involved.

Mediterranean Diet: Sun, Sea, and Olive Oil

First up, we have the Mediterranean Diet — a perennial favorite among health nuts and people who enjoy the occasional vacation to the Mediterranean (you know who you are).

What It Is: The Mediterranean Diet is all about embracing whole, nutrient-dense foods like fruits, vegetables, legumes, nuts, seeds, and of course, fish. Healthy fats, particularly olive oil, are the stars of this show, and dairy and red meat make a more modest appearance. Think of it as the diet equivalent of living the good life — sunshine, fresh air, and the occasional glass of wine. It's not about strict rules or deprivation; it's more of a philosophy that celebrates balance and sustainability. That's why it's not just a trendy diet—it's a lifestyle. Whether you're prepping for a fancy dinner party or just making a quick lunch, the Mediterranean approach fits right in.

The Pros:

1. *Heart Health Hero:* With a focus on healthy fats (especially omega-3s from fish), the Mediterranean Diet is famous for lowering the risk of heart disease. Who wouldn't want to live longer while enjoying delicious meals that keep their heart in tip-top shape? Plus, olive oil is known for its anti-inflammatory properties, which is basically like giving your insides a spa day.

2. *No Counting Calories*: One of the best parts? You don't need to count every calorie that passes your lips. Instead, the focus is on filling your plate with nutrient-rich, whole foods and eating in moderation. You'll feel good about what you're eating, and you won't need to bust out the calculator every time you snack. The Mediterranean Diet encourages balance—not perfection.

3. *Delicious and Sustainable:* If you've ever dreamed of eating like a Roman emperor (minus the empire collapse), this diet will make you feel like royalty. Fresh, flavorful meals that are easy on the eyes and even easier to enjoy. Whether it's a Mediterranean salad, grilled fish, or a simple plate of roasted vegetables, this diet serves up meals you'll actually look forward to. Plus, the emphasis on plant-based foods helps keep things light and vibrant, making it a sustainable choice for the long haul.

The Cons:

1. *Expensive Taste:* As much as we'd love to live like the rich and famous, eating fresh fish, high-quality olive oil, and plenty of nuts isn't cheap. Your grocery bill may start looking like

you're feeding a small army of seafaring adventurers. If you're on a budget, you may want to prepare yourself for a few extra trips to the bank before that shopping cart is full of Mediterranean goodness.

2. *Dairy Dilemma:* While this diet allows for some dairy — mainly in the form of cheese and yogurt — it's not an all-you-can-eat cheese buffet. For those who love their dairy with reckless abandon (hello, cheese addicts), the Mediterranean Diet may feel a little restrictive. Sorry, no mozzarella mountains or endless cheese platters at your next dinner party.

Mediterranean Diet is a flavorful and heart-healthy way of eating that emphasizes balance, fresh ingredients, and moderation. While it may come with a price tag and the occasional cheese withdrawal, it's a lifestyle that's as sustainable as it is delicious. So go ahead — sip that glass of red wine, drizzle some olive oil on your salad, and feel like you're on vacation, even if you're just at home.

Keto Diet: Fat, But Make It Fabulous

Now, we've entered the land of high fat and low carbs. Welcome to the world of ketosis, where your body starts burning fat instead of carbs as its primary fuel source. Are you ready to say goodbye to bread forever? Spoiler alert: not forever.

What It Is: The Keto Diet is all about drastically reducing carbs and increasing your fat intake to the point where your body enters a state called ketosis. In ketosis, your body starts breaking down fat into ketones, which then become your new energy source. This diet is a favorite among people looking to shed some pounds quickly, and it's also been used for managing conditions like epilepsy and Alzheimer's disease. So, if you're into the idea of burning fat like a well-oiled machine, this might just be the diet for you.

The Pros:

1. *Weight Loss, Baby:* Keto is like a turbo boost for fat burning. When done correctly, it forces your body to enter fat-burning mode and say goodbye to those pesky carbs. The result? Weight loss. It's like a personal trainer who's always there, nudging you to keep going (but without the motivational speech).

2. *Stable Energy:* Ever feel like you're riding a rollercoaster of energy highs and crashes throughout the day? Well, in ketosis, your body burns fat consistently for fuel, which means no more 3 p.m. slumps or mid-morning sugar crashes. You'll enjoy a more stable energy supply, which is kind of like upgrading from a go-kart to a sleek sports car.

3. *Mental Clarity:* Some keto devotees swear they experience mental clarity and focus once their body adapts to this new way of eating. It's as though your brain gets a fresh coat of paint—clearer and more focused. No more fuzzy thinking, just laser-sharp attention. It's like your brain's been to a spa, minus the carbs that tend to make you sluggish and foggy.

The Cons:

1. *Goodbye, Pasta: Now, the downside:* if you love bread, pasta, and rice, this diet will feel like a cruel punishment. Keto takes those carb-heavy foods and locks them in a cage, never to see the light of day again. It's like being asked to live in a world without your favorite TV shows—it's tough, and you might cry a little.

2. *Keto Flu:* In the early stages of keto, many people experience the "keto flu." It's a temporary mix of headaches, fatigue, nausea, and irritability. So, if you find yourself snapping at your friends or craving a massive bowl of spaghetti, don't blame them—blame it on ketosis and give it time to work its magic.

The Keto Diet is a powerful way to lose weight and boost energy by cutting carbs and embracing fat. But it's not all sunshine and rainbows—saying goodbye to pasta and enduring keto flu might make you question your life choices. Still, if you're up for the challenge, ketosis could be your ticket to a slimmer, more energized you. Just don't expect to see pasta again anytime soon.

Calorie Deficit: The Simple Science of Weight Loss

Let's talk about the not-so-secret formula for shedding fat: calorie deficit. No fancy diets, no complicated rules—just basic math. If you burn more calories than you consume, your body starts dipping into its fat stores for energy, and voilà—you lose weight. Sounds easy, right? Well, there's a bit more to it, but that's the core principle.

What It Is: A calorie deficit happens when the number of calories you consume is lower than the number of calories you burn. Think of it like budgeting, but for your body. If your daily calorie requirement is 2000 calories, but you only eat 1500, your body has to make up for that missing 500 calories by burning stored fat. Add some exercise into the mix, and you can increase your deficit, leading to even more fat loss. It's like making your body work extra hard to "find" fuel, and guess where it looks first? Those stubborn fat stores.

The Pros:

1. Effective for Weight Loss – No matter what diet trend is in the spotlight, weight loss always comes down to one thing: a calorie deficit. Whether you're doing keto, intermittent fasting, or just eating healthier, if you're not in a deficit, you won't lose weight. It's science.

2. No Food Restrictions – Unlike other diets that cut out entire food groups (*goodbye, carbs*), calorie deficit doesn't tell you

what to eat—it just tells you how much. Want a slice of pizza? Cool, just fit it into your daily calorie limit. Balance is key!

3. Boosts Metabolism (When Done Right) - A moderate deficit encourages your body to burn fat efficiently while keeping your metabolism steady. You'll feel lighter, more energetic, and less sluggish throughout the day.

The Cons:

1. Portion Control Reality Check - You quickly realize that some foods are *calorie bombs*. A single fast-food meal can take up your entire day's worth of calories. Cue the heartbreak. Learning to portion control and make smarter choices is crucial.

2. Too Much Deficit = Trouble - If you go too extreme (like eating 800 calories a day), your body flips into survival mode, slows metabolism, and holds onto fat instead. The result? You feel exhausted, cranky, and your weight loss stalls. No fun.

3. Exercise is Optional but Recommended - You can lose weight just by eating less, but adding workouts helps speed things up. Plus, strength training ensures that you lose fat *instead* of muscle, keeping you strong and toned.

Calorie deficit is the foundation of weight loss—no gimmicks, no magic pills, just burning more than you eat. The key is to create a sustainable deficit that fits your lifestyle. Make smart food choices, watch portions, and move your body. Whether you want to lose 5 or 50 pounds, this is *the* strategy that actually works.

Paleo Diet: Eating Like a Caveman (Without the Cave)

Next up, we've got the Paleo Diet, which is essentially the ultimate "throwback" diet. Think of it as going back in time and eating like your caveman ancestors. No processed foods, no grains, just whole, natural foods. Who knew cavemen had such good taste?

What It Is: The Paleo Diet is based on the premise that humans should eat like our ancient ancestors. That means lean meats, fish, fruits, vegetables, nuts, and seeds — basically, anything that can be foraged, hunted, or gathered. Forget about dairy, grains, legumes, and processed foods. If it wasn't around during the Paleolithic era, it's not allowed on the menu. So, if you ever wanted an excuse to eat like a hunter-gatherer and show off your primal side, now's your chance! Just don't expect to dig into a bowl of pasta or cake. If dessert is a must for you, you'll need to get creative. Spoiler alert: fruit is about as sweet as it gets.

The Pros:

1. *Whole Foods Galore:* The Paleo Diet emphasizes nutrient-dense, whole foods. No processed junk — just good, clean eating. It's like the food version of spring cleaning for your body. Plus, you'll be packing in loads of vitamins, minerals, and healthy fats from natural sources. Say goodbye to that bag of chips and hello to a better, more vibrant you.

2. *Weight Loss Potential:* Since it cuts out processed foods and focuses on clean, whole foods, the Paleo Diet can lead to weight loss. When your meals are primarily made up of lean meats, vegetables, and healthy fats, you'll feel fuller for longer and be less likely to snack on unhealthy foods. But, just to clarify, you won't be dropping pounds while binge-watching Netflix and pretending to be a caveman in your living room.

3. *Blood Sugar Control:* The Paleo Diet eliminates refined sugars and processed foods, which can help stabilize blood sugar levels. This makes it a great choice for people managing diabetes or those looking to avoid blood sugar spikes. You

won't be relying on that mid-afternoon sugar rush—just steady, natural energy throughout the day.

The Cons:

1. *No Grains, No Fun:* One of the biggest challenges of the Paleo Diet is that grains are off-limits. That means no pasta, rice, bread, or even quinoa (yes, we're crying too). If your soul is entwined with pizza or sandwiches, this might be a tough pill to swallow. And let's not even talk about croissants. They don't exist in Paleo land.

2. *Expensive:* Fresh, high-quality meats, vegetables, and wild-caught fish aren't exactly cheap. If you're sticking to the Paleo lifestyle long-term, you might need to budget like a pro. You'll be looking at your grocery bill and thinking, "Did I just buy a whole herd of bison?" That said, investing in quality foods now could pay off in the long run by supporting your health and well-being.

So, there you have it. The Paleo Diet is all about returning to basics with nutrient-dense, whole foods. While it offers health benefits like weight loss and blood sugar control, it does come with some challenges, like bidding farewell to your favorite carbs and shelling out some extra cash for groceries. If you're up for channeling your inner caveman, it might just be the diet for you!

Vegan Diet: Save the Planet, One Tofu Stir-Fry at a Time

Now we enter the world of plant-based living. If you're looking to be as kind to the planet as possible while also not eating anything that ever had a heartbeat, the Vegan Diet might be for you. It's like taking a stand for the Earth and its inhabitants, one avocado toast at a time.

What It Is: The Vegan Diet is all about excluding all animal products. No meat, no dairy, no eggs—nothing that ever came from a creature that once had a heartbeat. Instead, you'll be focusing on plant-based foods—fruits, vegetables, grains, legumes, nuts, seeds, and plant-based proteins (think tofu, tempeh, and seitan). Some people choose this lifestyle for ethical reasons (animal rights, anyone?), others because of environmental concerns, and a few do it for health reasons, hoping to score some major wellness benefits. Regardless of the motivation, veganism is as green as it gets—and we mean that in both the ethical and literal sense (hello, green veggies!).

The Pros:

1. *Animal Lover's Dream*: If you're passionate about animal rights, the Vegan Diet is like the ultimate expression of your values. No cows, pigs, chickens, or fish need to be involved in your meal prep. If you've ever watched an animal documentary and thought, "I can't keep supporting that," this is your golden ticket to a more compassionate lifestyle.

2. *Weight Loss and Health Benefits:* A well-balanced vegan diet can help with weight loss by reducing your intake of unhealthy fats and cholesterol that often come with animal products. More fruits and veggies mean more fiber, vitamins, and minerals, giving you that health glow without the guilt of a greasy burger.

3. *Heart Health:* Since vegan diets tend to be lower in saturated fats and cholesterol, they're heart-friendly. Plus, a diet rich in plant-based foods is often associated with lower risks of heart disease and high blood pressure. More fiber, less fat—sounds like a win for your heart and arteries!

The Cons:

1. *You Miss Cheese, Don't You?:* Let's face it, if you love cheese, transitioning to a vegan lifestyle is like learning to live without your childhood friend. You know, the one who was

always there for you during late-night study sessions and pizza parties? Yeah, vegan cheese doesn't always hit the same spot (though there are some amazing options if you dig deep enough, so hang in there).

2. *Nutrient Gaps:* While a vegan diet is rich in fruits, vegetables, and whole grains, it can sometimes fall short in nutrients like B12, iron, and omega-3 fatty acids. These nutrients are typically found in animal products, so if you're not careful, you might find yourself running on empty. Make sure to supplement as needed to avoid deficiencies and keep your energy up.

The Vegan Diet is a great option for those who want to align their eating habits with their ethical, environmental, and health goals. But, if you're not ready to say goodbye to cheese forever, or if you're concerned about nutrient gaps, it might take some adjusting. The journey to plant-based living is full of tofu, tempeh, and an occasional (sorrowful) goodbye to cheese.

DASH Diet: Eating for Your Blood Pressure

The DASH (Dietary Approaches to Stop Hypertension) Diet is a go-to for people looking to keep their blood pressure in check and avoid becoming a human stress ball. If you're aiming for a diet that promotes heart health without major sacrifices or cutting out entire food groups, this one might just be your new best friend.

What It Is: The DASH Diet is focused on foods rich in potassium, calcium, magnesium, and fiber. Think of it as the diet that helps keep your heart healthy and your blood pressure in check. It emphasizes eating fruits, vegetables, whole grains, lean proteins, and low-fat dairy while cutting down on sodium, sugar, and red meat. The goal is to reduce the risk of hypertension (high blood pressure) and improve overall cardiovascular health. Unlike other diets that require extreme cuts or restrictions, DASH is about making healthier, sustainable food choices.

The Pros:

1. *Blood Pressure Friendly:* The DASH Diet is specifically designed to lower high blood pressure. With its emphasis on potassium and magnesium-rich foods like bananas, leafy greens, and beans, it acts like a delicious prescription for heart health. By reducing sodium and incorporating heart-healthy nutrients, it helps keep blood pressure levels within a normal range, which reduces the risk of heart disease and stroke.

2. *Easy to Follow*: Unlike many restrictive diets, DASH doesn't involve cutting out entire food groups. You won't find yourself yearning for a forbidden food item because you can still enjoy a balanced diet, including whole grains, fruits, vegetables, and lean proteins. It's a lot more flexible than many other diets that might require complicated meal plans or highly specific food lists.

3. *Overall Health Boost:* The DASH Diet doesn't just lower blood pressure. Studies suggest that it may help prevent heart disease, strokes, kidney stones, and even some cancers. The combination of nutrient-rich foods supports your body's overall health, making it a great long-term lifestyle change. You're not just eating to manage one issue—you're giving your body a full health boost.

The Cons:

1. *Not Always Instant Results:* The DASH Diet isn't about rapid weight loss. It may take some time to see significant results in terms of lowering your blood pressure or shedding pounds. So, if you're looking for a quick fix, this might feel like a slower path compared to diets that promise fast results.

2. *High on Whole Foods*: DASH emphasizes whole, fresh foods, which means you'll need to do some cooking and meal prepping. If you're someone who loves convenience or relies

heavily on takeout, this might require a shift in your routine. It's a diet that calls for investment in fresh ingredients and a bit of time in the kitchen.

DASH Diet is an excellent option for those seeking a heart-healthy, sustainable approach to eating that supports blood pressure management and overall well-being. If you're ready for a longer-term commitment to your health with fewer sacrifices, DASH might be just what you need.

Whole30 Diet: The 30-Day Reset (That Feels Like Forever)

Whole30 is the 30-day elimination diet where you cut out sugar, alcohol, grains, dairy, legumes, and processed foods to reset your eating habits. Think of it as the tough-love approach to clean eating—taking a deep dive into healthy eating by eliminating potentially inflammatory foods and foods you might not realize are causing problems.

What It Is: Whole30 is all about taking a break from common food triggers to help identify sensitivities and reset your relationship with food. For a full 30 days, you eliminate sugar, alcohol, grains, legumes, dairy, and processed foods, and focus on whole, nutrient-dense options like meat, vegetables, fruits, and healthy fats. The idea is that by the end of the month, your cravings will be more in line with healthy eating, and you'll have a better understanding of which foods are making you feel sluggish, bloated, or unwell.

The Pros:

1. *A Complete Reset:* If you've been living off takeout or indulging in too many processed foods, Whole30 offers a chance for a clean slate. This is your opportunity to reset your cravings and start fresh with whole foods that fuel your body. After the 30 days, you might find you have a clearer mind, more energy, and better digestion.

2. *Increased Awareness:* One of the main benefits of Whole30 is that it helps you tune into how specific foods make you feel. After cutting out common inflammatory foods, you'll have a chance to reintroduce them one by one to see which ones cause bloating, fatigue, or other reactions. It can make you more mindful about what you eat long-term, promoting healthier choices after the challenge ends.
3. *Discipline and Clean Eating:* Whole30 encourages you to cook from scratch and rely on whole, unprocessed foods. It helps build discipline in your eating habits and teaches you how to prepare meals that nourish your body and help you feel your best.

The Cons:

1. *A Whole Lotta No:* The first challenge you'll face is the number of food restrictions. You're saying no to grains, legumes, dairy, and alcohol for a full 30 days. If you love your morning coffee with milk, a slice of pizza, or a glass of wine, you might feel like you're living in a food prison.
2. *Strict and Socially Challenging:* Whole30 isn't just hard to maintain in your everyday routine; it can be socially isolating. Eating out, attending parties, or social gatherings can become tricky when most foods are off-limits. You'll have to exercise willpower and possibly explain your diet to confused friends and family.

In short, Whole30 is a great tool if you're looking for a reset, but it's not for the faint of heart. It's a strict diet, designed to help you reset your habits and identify potential food sensitivities, but the restrictions might leave you feeling deprived at times. If you're up for the challenge, Whole30 can be a great way to start a new, healthier chapter.

Low-Carb Diet: Fewer Carbs, More Problems?

The low-carb diet is a popular eating plan that focuses on reducing carbohydrates (like pasta, bread, and sugar) while emphasizing proteins and fats. By cutting back on carbs, the body shifts to burning fat for energy, which can result in rapid weight loss and other health benefits. Think Atkins or similar plans that let you say goodbye to those carb-heavy meals and hello to a higher protein and fat intake.

What It Is: Low-carb diets typically involve reducing carb consumption and replacing those calories with proteins and healthy fats. This approach encourages the body to enter a state where it uses fat for energy rather than carbohydrates. Popular versions of the low-carb diet include the Atkins Diet, Keto, and other similar plans. While they vary in the extent of carb restriction, they all share the goal of limiting carbs, particularly refined ones like white bread, pasta, and sugary foods.

The Pros:

1. *Rapid Weight Loss:* One of the biggest draws of the low-carb diet is its potential for fast weight loss. In the initial stages, the body burns through stored carbohydrates (glycogen) and water weight, which leads to rapid weight loss. Over time, the body switches to burning fat for fuel, helping with sustained weight loss. Many people report seeing quicker results than with other diets.

2. *Blood Sugar Regulation:* Low-carb diets can help regulate blood sugar levels, which is beneficial for people with diabetes or those at risk of developing diabetes. By limiting carbohydrate intake, especially refined sugars, the body has a more stable insulin response, helping avoid spikes in blood sugar.

3. *Improved Heart Health:* By increasing the intake of healthy fats and proteins, a low-carb diet may help improve heart health.

Reducing the consumption of processed carbs can lower the risk of heart disease by reducing inflammation and improving cholesterol levels.

The Cons:

1. *Limited Food Options:* One of the main downsides of the low-carb diet is the limited range of foods available. Many people miss out on beloved carbs like bread, pasta, rice, and even certain fruits. For carb lovers, this can feel restrictive, making the diet hard to stick to in the long term.

2. *Possible Nutrient Gaps:* By cutting out carbs, you might miss out on essential vitamins and minerals, particularly those found in whole grains, fruits, and vegetables. A lack of fiber, vitamins (like vitamin C), and other nutrients can lead to deficiencies over time if not carefully managed.

A low-carb diet can offer rapid weight loss, better blood sugar control, and even heart health benefits, but it comes with some challenges. Limited food choices and the potential for nutrient gaps can make it a difficult lifestyle to maintain. If you're considering this diet, it's essential to plan carefully to ensure you get a well-rounded, nutrient-dense diet while minimizing the carb intake.

Intermittent Fasting: The Art of Skipping Breakfast (On Purpose)

Let's talk about intermittent fasting (IF), the "skip meals and still be healthy" diet that has captured the attention of millions. It's not about what you eat but when you eat—an intriguing concept, right? Get ready to break the cycle of three meals a day and embrace fasting windows that could lead to weight loss and other health benefits.

What It Is: Intermittent fasting involves alternating between periods of eating and fasting. The most common method is the 16/8 approach, where you fast for 16 hours (yes, that includes sleeping!)

and eat within an 8-hour window. So, if you finish dinner at 8 p.m., your next meal could be at noon the following day. Another version includes fasting for 24 hours once or twice a week. The core idea is that it's less about the food you eat and more about when you eat it—allowing your body to switch gears and burn fat instead of constantly digesting food.

The Pros:

1. Weight Loss Wizard: One of the most appealing aspects of intermittent fasting is its weight loss potential. By reducing the eating window, you're naturally likely to eat fewer calories. Plus, IF helps regulate insulin levels, which in turn encourages your body to burn fat during the fasting periods. It's a simpler way to shed pounds without counting every calorie, which makes it easier to stick to.

2. Improved Metabolism: Some studies suggest that intermittent fasting can improve metabolism and even increase longevity. By giving your digestive system a break and boosting fat-burning processes, IF can contribute to a healthier metabolism. Who wouldn't want to live longer with more energy?

3. Mental Clarity: When you're fasting, your body goes into a heightened state of alertness. This means many people report feeling sharper and more focused during fasting periods. Imagine being mentally clear and productive—without the carb crash or post-meal sluggishness.

The Cons:

1. *Hunger Pangs*: If you're a die-hard breakfast fan, intermittent fasting might be a tough pill to swallow. Skipping that first meal of the day can lead to serious hunger pangs, making it hard to stick with the plan, especially in the beginning. The first few fasting days can feel like an exercise in self-control.

2. *Social Challenges:* Socializing while fasting can be a bit awkward. If your fasting window happens to coincide with when your friends or family want to eat, you'll have to explain why you're not joining in. Playing the "I'm fasting, please don't judge me" card can be uncomfortable, especially if they're tucking into your favorite food.

Intermittent fasting offers a simple way to regulate your eating habits, lose weight, and possibly gain mental clarity and better metabolism. But if you're not ready to skip breakfast or deal with social challenges, it might take a bit of practice to make it work for you.

Time Restricted Eating (TRE) and Time Restricted Fasting (TRF): A Deep Dive with a Dash of Humor

In the world of diets, Time Restricted Eating (TRE) and Time Restricted Fasting (TRF) have become the "cool kids on the block," gaining popularity for their simplicity and potential health benefits. These eating patterns revolve around one very straightforward idea: it's not just about what you eat—it's about *when* you eat. Let's break it down with a sprinkle of humor, because hey, a healthy lifestyle doesn't have to be all serious business.

What Is Time Restricted Eating (TRE)?

Time Restricted Eating (TRE) is like giving your body a very organized, punctual work schedule. TRE involves eating all your meals within a specific window of time during the day, and fasting for the rest. Imagine it like a strict office hours schedule for your stomach. A common pattern is the 16/8 method, where you fast for 16 hours (including your beauty sleep) and eat during an 8-hour window. That's right—no breakfast, but hey, you get to enjoy lunch and dinner without guilt.

The beauty of TRE is that it's all about *timing*, not so much *restriction*. You can eat whatever you want (well, within reason) as long as it fits within your designated eating window. So go ahead, enjoy that avocado toast or those tacos—just not at 7 a.m., unless you're in the 8-hour window. It's about managing the timing of your meals and letting your body process food more effectively, burning fat during the fasting periods, and keeping you feeling energetic.

What Is Time Restricted Fasting (TRF)?

Time Restricted Fasting (TRF) is like TRE's cooler, more intense cousin. TRF is essentially an eating pattern where you fast for a longer stretch of time, often around 14 to 20 hours. It's like TRE but with a little more *kick*—you're fasting for longer and eating for a shorter period. If TRE is like a chill stroll through the park, TRF is more of a "let's climb that mountain" type of deal. An example is the 18/6 method, where you eat within a 6-hour window (say 12 p.m. to 6 p.m.) and fast for the remaining 18 hours.

TRF is all about giving your body time to reset and repair. Think of it as an opportunity for your body to hit the "refresh" button. You know, like when your computer is running slow and you restart it? TRF is essentially your body doing a full reboot, burning fat, improving metabolism, and giving your digestive system some much-needed time off. It's like a spa day for your insides.

Benefits of Time Restricted Eating and Time Restricted Fasting

Both TRE and TRF have some pretty awesome benefits, and unlike most diets, they don't require you to spend hours measuring your food or cutting out entire food groups. Here's why you might want to give it a shot:

1. *Improved Metabolic Health:* When you're fasting, your body has more time to process glucose, improving insulin sensitivity. Think of it as your body getting better at its job,

like when you finally organize your closet and things stop falling out every time you open the door.

2. *Weight Loss and Fat Burning:* Both TRE and TRF encourage your body to burn fat instead of carbs during fasting. It's like telling your body, "Okay, time to start burning those stored snacks you've been hoarding."

3. *Cellular Repair and Longevity:* Fasting helps trigger autophagy, which is your body's way of cleaning out damaged cells and regenerating new ones. It's like giving your body a little tune-up so it can run like a well-oiled machine for years to come.

4. *Increased Mental Clarity:* During fasting, many people report feeling sharper and more focused. It's like your brain is finally getting the memo: "Let's stop clouding up with food distractions and get to work!"

5. *Gut Health and Digestion:* Giving your digestive system a break can work wonders for gut health. It's like telling your stomach, "You've been working hard, so take a well-deserved nap."

6. *Simplified Eating Routine:* If you're tired of meal prepping for hours, TRE and TRF offer a simpler approach. You eat within a set window, and that's it. No need for complicated meal plans—just a little food, a little timing, and boom, you're done.

Timing is Everything: TRE, TRF, and Your Circadian Rhythm

We often focus on *what* we eat, but *when* we eat is just as important. Our bodies function on a natural internal clock called the circadian rhythm, which controls everything from sleep cycles to metabolism. This 24-hour cycle is influenced by light, darkness, and even meal timing. When we eat in sync with our circadian rhythm, we optimize digestion, energy levels, and even fat loss.

This is where Time-Restricted Eating (TRE) and Time-Restricted Feeding (TRF) come in. Both methods focus on eating within a specific window of time and fasting for the rest of the day. Unlike traditional diets that obsess over calorie counting, TRE and TRF work with your body's natural rhythm, allowing you to eat in a way that enhances metabolism, balances hormones, and improves overall health.

Your metabolism isn't static; it changes throughout the day. In the morning, your body is primed for digestion, energy production, and fat burning. As the day winds down, so does your metabolism, making late-night eating a recipe for sluggish digestion and weight gain. TRE and TRF work by syncing your meals with your body's most efficient metabolic phases, ensuring you're burning fuel at the right times and not storing excess energy as fat.

By incorporating these methods into your routine, you're not just following another diet—you're optimizing your body's natural clock for long-term health benefits.

Now that we've covered how meal timing influences metabolism, it's time to dive deeper into the circadian rhythm itself. From regulating sleep to controlling hunger hormones, this internal clock plays a crucial role in how we function daily. Understanding how to align your lifestyle with your circadian rhythm can be a game-changer for weight management, energy levels, and overall well-being.

Pick Your Poison (Or Not)

In the end, choosing the right diet boils down to one simple truth: it's about finding what works for you. Whether you're drawn to the balanced approach of a plant-based diet, the high-protein focus of carnivore eating, or the structured discipline of intermittent fasting, there's no one-size-fits-all solution. The key to long-term success isn't just about what's on your plate—it's about how seamlessly a diet fits into your lifestyle. Are you willing to track macros like a scientist, or do you prefer a more intuitive approach that lets you enjoy food without overthinking every bite?

Some diets focus on metabolic flexibility, like carb cycling, which alternates between high- and low-carb days to optimize energy and fat loss. Others, like intermittent fasting, use meal timing to tap into fat-burning mode while giving digestion a break. And if you thrive on simplicity, the Paleo diet's back-to-basics philosophy may be your best bet. But no matter what approach you choose — whether it's cutting carbs, eating more protein, or timing your meals strategically — it all comes down to one thing: how you feel.

The trick to dietary success is sustainability. Short-term results are great, but if a diet leaves you constantly exhausted, miserable, or obsessing over that forbidden slice of cake, it's probably not the best fit. No eating plan is perfect, and each one has its own challenges. But with a little planning, flexibility, and a sense of humor, any diet can be enjoyable — yes, even the ones that seem restrictive at first. Whether you're structuring your day around protein-packed meals, experimenting with fasting, or simply making an effort to eat more whole foods, the goal is to create a lifestyle that supports your health without feeling like a punishment.

The best diet isn't just about the food — it's about how it aligns with your body's natural rhythms. Timing your meals properly, understanding when and how much to eat, and choosing foods that work *with* your metabolism instead of against it can make all the difference.

This is why I personally follow a structure based on circadian rhythm principles — a natural way of eating that optimizes digestion, energy, and overall health. Keeping this in mind, here's what my daily eating pattern looks like. If it seems doable for you, I highly recommend giving it a try to bring your lifestyle into a smooth, effortless flow.

If you're wondering whether a particular diet is worth committing to, remember this: no choice is permanent. No way of eating should feel like a life sentence. The beauty of nutrition is that you have the freedom to experiment and adjust as you go. Pick your poison—or not—but most importantly, focus on what fuels your body best.

Understanding the Circadian Rhythm – The Body's Natural Clock

Alright, let's talk about something that governs every single one of us without us even realizing it—our body's *internal clock*. Now, I know what you're thinking: "Wait, I don't have an actual clock inside me—what is this sorcery?" But trust me, you do! It's called your circadian rhythm, and it's basically the ultimate time manager for your body. Think of it as the most reliable (and persistent) boss who insists on keeping you in sync with the world around you — whether you like it or not.

The circadian rhythm is a 24-hour cycle that plays a starring role in regulating pretty much every essential process in your body, from when you wake up to when you go to sleep. It's like the conductor of a symphony, making sure your body functions in harmony with the world. It tells you when to feel sleepy, when to wake up, and how to keep your digestion running smoothly. Yes, it even affects your hormones—those pesky little molecules that seem to dictate your mood, energy, and appetite. The circadian rhythm literally controls when you should be hungry (and when you shouldn't reach for that extra donut).

Here's where it gets a little tricky, though. Your circadian rhythm doesn't just run on auto-pilot—no, no, it's deeply influenced by the natural rhythms of the environment around you. The rising and setting of the sun, light exposure, temperature changes—your internal clock is constantly listening to these cues. It's as though your body's very own orchestra is trying to play its best tune, but it needs the environment to be in sync for everything to sound just right.

Now, when your body is working in perfect sync with the rhythms of nature, you feel like a rockstar. You wake up feeling refreshed, energized, and ready to take on the day (even if it's just getting through a never-ending Zoom call). But when that internal clock gets out of sync — say, you pull an all-nighter or you're staring at your phone in bed past midnight — things start to unravel. It's like the orchestra going completely out of tune. Suddenly, your digestion is off, your energy crashes at the wrong times, and you might feel like you've been hit by a bus (that bus being sleep deprivation).

That's why syncing your circadian rhythm with the natural world is so crucial for your health. It's not just a matter of feeling a little off after a late-night binge-watching session (though, that's certainly a side effect). If your circadian rhythm gets too out of whack, it can mess with your hormones, your immune system, and even increase your risk of developing some pretty serious health issues. So, if you're hoping to be the best version of yourself — physically, mentally, and emotionally — it's time to listen to your body's clock and get in tune with the rhythm of nature.

The good news? There are simple, easy ways to reset and realign with your body's internal clock. You don't need to throw out your alarm clock (though, let's be honest, that thing's probably an unwelcome guest anyway). Just a little understanding of your circadian rhythm and a few changes to your daily habits can help you get back on track — and that's where we come in. Welcome to the world of circadian harmony!

What is the Circadian Rhythm?

Alright, folks, let's get down to the basics. The *circadian rhythm* sounds pretty fancy, doesn't it? But, in reality, it's just a big ol' 24-hour cycle that runs all of the body's important processes. Think of it like the world's most punctual and diligent project manager. It ensures that everything in your body runs on time—sleep, digestion, hormone release—you name it. If you've ever wondered why you feel like a night owl at 3 AM but could fall into a coma by 9 PM, your circadian rhythm is the culprit, controlling when you should sleep, eat, or even feel most energetic. It's the ultimate natural timekeeper, and it doesn't take a day off.

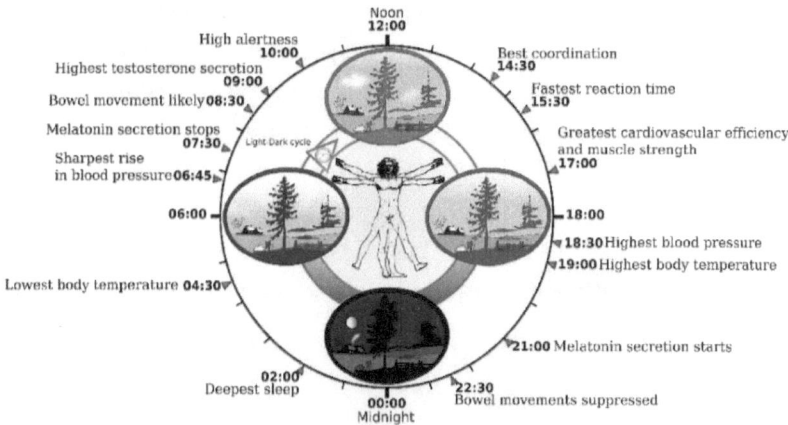

Now, where did this idea of a circadian rhythm even come from? Let's take a little stroll down history lane, shall we? Scientists first stumbled upon this rhythm back in the 1950s when they realized that living organisms seemed to follow a consistent pattern of activity and rest over a 24-hour period. It wasn't just a coincidence that we were waking up with the sunrise and falling asleep around sunset—it was our bodies aligning with the natural world. You see, it's no accident that we sleep at night and wake up when it's light out. It's all part of a beautiful, perfectly timed biological choreography.

But wait, there's more! It wasn't until the 1960s that scientists discovered the real boss of this whole operation: the *master clock*. This genius timekeeper resides in your brain's hypothalamus—sounds important, right? The hypothalamus is like your body's personal headquarters, and it controls this entire circadian rhythm operation. This master clock gets its cues from the environment, primarily from light and dark cycles. So when you're exposed to light in the morning, it signals to your brain that it's time to wake up and be fabulous. When the evening rolls in, and darkness sets in, it cues your body to wind down and get some rest. Essentially, your hypothalamus is the CEO, and everything else is working to keep the rhythm in check.

But here's the twist—there's not just one clock in your body. Oh no. Your circadian rhythm's influence spreads throughout various biological systems, like a CEO with multiple companies. Each organ or system in your body has its own smaller biological clock. For example, your sleep-wake cycle, metabolism, immune response, and even mood are all influenced by your circadian rhythm. It's like having a bunch of tiny employees spread throughout your body, all working in perfect harmony (most of the time, anyway).

Let's break it down further:

- Sleep: Your body is programmed to feel sleepy at night and awake during the day, thanks to the circadian rhythm. Without it, you'd probably fall asleep while eating lunch or feel wide-eyed and bushy-tailed at 2 AM.
- Metabolism: Your digestive system knows when to work its hardest, based on the rhythm. Ever notice how you're starving right when you wake up? That's your metabolism kicking into high gear as it knows it's time to process food.
- Mood: Your circadian rhythm also affects your serotonin levels, which is why you might feel like a grump without your morning coffee or sunny weather. On cloudy days, you may feel a little more sluggish—blame your internal clock for that too!

- Immune response: Turns out, your immune system isn't a 24/7 worker either. It takes cues from your circadian rhythm, working harder during the day to protect you from threats and doing some "maintenance" while you sleep.

So there you have it—your circadian rhythm is like a little maestro conducting the symphony of your life. It's what makes you feel sleepy, alert, hungry, and even happy at the right times. And believe me, you *do not* want to upset this rhythm—it's the one thing keeping you from turning into a cranky, zombie-like version of yourself.

The Science Behind the Circadian Rhythm

Okay, let's get a little more scientific, shall we? Don't worry, I'll keep it fun. You see, when it comes to your body's timekeeping system, the *hypothalamus* is like the conductor of an orchestra—except instead of music, it's your internal clock keeping everything in sync. You've probably heard of the hypothalamus before—it's that little brain region that gets a bad rap for managing all the "boring" stuff like hunger, thirst, and body temperature regulation. But here's the thing: it's also the *master* of your body's time system.

So, what's going on inside this tiny-but-mighty region? The hypothalamus houses the *suprachiasmatic nucleus* (SCN)—say that three times fast—your body's official "timekeeper." The SCN is responsible for regulating your circadian rhythm by receiving light signals from your eyes and adjusting your internal processes accordingly. Imagine the SCN as your body's personal smartphone alarm clock, except instead of beeping obnoxiously, it uses light cues to wake you up and put you to sleep. It's like waking up to sunshine rather than an alarm ringing in your ear. Who wouldn't want that?

Now, what's the deal with *light*? Turns out, light is like the VIP guest in your circadian rhythm party. The SCN reacts to natural light exposure during the day and uses that signal to keep track of time. When the sun rises and your eyes are exposed to natural light (hello, morning sunlight!), the SCN gets the memo: "Okay, time to kick things into high gear. Let's get this person awake and alert." But when it's dark, the SCN tells your body, "Alright, folks, time to slow down and prepare for some much-needed rest." It's the ultimate reminder that nature has your back when it comes to your sleep-wake cycle.

And here's the kicker: light is also responsible for resetting your circadian rhythm, which is why getting some good sunlight in the morning is key to staying in sync. So, if you've been struggling to fall asleep or feel groggy all day, your rhythm might be a little out of whack. Trust me, your circadian rhythm is just waiting for you to be a little more consistent with your exposure to natural light.

Now, let's talk hormones. Hormones are the drama queens of the body. They make things happen, they disrupt things, and they absolutely love to follow their own schedule. The most famous circadian rhythm duo is *cortisol* and *melatonin* — both of whom work in tandem to regulate your sleep-wake cycle.

Cortisol, often known as the "stress hormone," is also your *morning hero*. It's responsible for making sure you wake up feeling alert, ready to conquer the day (or at least get out of bed without feeling like a zombie). The catch? Your cortisol levels should be *higher* in the morning and *lower* by nightfall. So if you're feeling like a grumpy sloth at night, blame it on cortisol not winding down properly.

Then there's melatonin, the *sleep hormone* — the one who's all about making sure you actually sleep like a peaceful baby. As the sun sets, your body starts pumping melatonin out like it's going out of style, signaling to your brain that it's time to wind down and sleep. Unfortunately, if your circadian rhythm is out of sync (thanks to late-night Netflix binges or scrolling through your phone in the dark), your melatonin production gets all messed up. And that's when the sleepless nights begin.

So, to wrap it all up: light exposure during the day sets the stage for your body to release cortisol in the morning (to make sure you don't hit the snooze button all day) and melatonin at night (so you can sleep like a baby). But if you're messing with your rhythm—hello, blue light from your phone at midnight—it can throw off these hormonal cues, leading to sleep troubles and mood swings. Remember: your body's internal clock may not always *feel* like a literal ticking watch, but it sure is the reason you feel awake, alert, or ready for bed at all the right times. Keep it in sync, and your body will thank you!

The Stages of the Circadian Rhythm and Their Impact on the Body

Ah, the circadian rhythm: It's like the internal playlist of your day. It starts with a wake-up jam, builds up to a peak performance rock anthem, winds down to a mellow evening tune, and finally, fades into a sleep lullaby. So, let's take a look at what happens throughout these stages and how they impact your body.

Morning (Wake-Up Phase)

You know that groggy, barely-open-eye feeling when you wake up? Yeah, that's because your body is still transitioning from dreamland. But then, like a superhero swooping in to save the day, *cortisol* enters the scene. Cortisol, also known as the "get-up-and-go" hormone, is responsible for helping you wake up and start your day. It's like your body's internal espresso shot—without the jitters.

To make the most of this phase, your body craves *sunlight*, and when you get a healthy dose of morning sunshine (the earlier, the better), you're helping your body adjust its internal clock. That sunlight tells your brain, "Alright, it's time to stop snoozing and start cruising." Getting that sunlight also boosts alertness and focus—basically, it's your secret weapon to fight off that early-morning fog. Plus, it improves energy levels and sets you up for a productive day ahead. So, next time you're tempted to stay in bed under the covers (we get it, it's cozy), remember that the sun is out there waiting to help you slay your day.

Afternoon (Peak Performance Phase)

Now, it's the *prime time* for your body, when your circadian rhythm is truly in sync with its peak performance. You'll feel like an absolute boss, mentally sharp, focused, and ready to take on the world. Seriously, this is when your body is like, "Let's crush some tasks!" Whether you're nailing that presentation or finishing up your to-do list, your body is at its prime. It's the *sweet spot* when you can go full throttle without burning out.

Your body also loves this time for exercise. So if you're trying to hit the gym or go for a run, this is your golden hour—your muscles are primed, and your energy is at its peak. Even better, eating meals in sync with your circadian rhythm (yes, that means lunch) helps boost digestion and keeps your energy steady throughout the afternoon. It's like filling up your tank with premium gas for a smooth ride.

Evening (Wind-Down Phase)

As the day winds down, your body starts to shift into relaxation mode. Cortisol, that early-morning energizer, starts to take a backseat, and *melatonin*, the "sleepy-time" hormone, starts to crank up the volume. This is when your body says, "Okay, we've had a productive day. Let's slow down and prepare for a good night's rest."

Now is when it's *crucial* to avoid those late-night Netflix binges (yes, we know you love that next episode) or scrolling through social media like it's a race to the finish line. The blue light from screens messes with melatonin production, and suddenly you're fighting your body's natural rhythm, wondering why you're wide awake at 2 a.m. So, instead of battling your internal clock, start relaxing with a good book, some calming music, or a warm cup of tea. Trust us, your future self will thank you.

Night (Sleep Phase)

Finally, it's time to rest, recharge, and hit that sweet spot where your body goes into sleep mode. The body's natural desire to sleep isn't just about *being tired*; it's about giving your body the chance to restore itself. Deep sleep works its magic during this phase — helping with physical repair, memory consolidation, and even detoxification. Yes, that means while you're blissfully unaware in your bed, your body is hard at work — so don't feel guilty about hitting that pillow.

A consistent sleep schedule is your golden ticket to maintaining harmony with your circadian rhythm. Going to bed and waking up at the same time each day helps keep things in sync, allowing your body to reset and recharge like the well-oiled machine it's meant to be.

So there you have it — your body's internal playlist. From the morning wake-up jam to the mellow wind-down evening ballad, syncing with your circadian rhythm is the key to feeling your best throughout the day. And hey, who doesn't want to wake up feeling like they can take on the world and wind down with a sense of calm, knowing a restful night's sleep is just around the corner?

The Impact of Disrupted Circadian Rhythms

Ah, the good old circadian rhythm — our body's internal clock that tells us when it's time to wake up, be productive, or take a nap (hello, 3 p.m. slump). But when that rhythm gets disrupted, oh boy, things can get messy. Whether you're pulling all-nighters, working odd shifts, or jetting across time zones like a professional traveler, messing with your internal clock is like trying to skip the opening credits of your favorite show—you're missing out on the crucial stuff.

Effects on Sleep

So, let's get to the heart of the matter: disrupted sleep. When you mess with your circadian rhythm, your body's natural sleep-wake cycle, you're asking for trouble. Shift work? Jet lag? Late-night Netflix marathons? All of these are prime culprits for wrecking your sleep, and boy, do they love to cause chaos. Instead of enjoying the bliss of deep, restorative sleep, you end up tossing and turning, battling an internal battle between your body's "it's time to sleep" signals and your mind's "hey, I just watched five episodes of *Stranger Things*—let's stay up all night!" signals.

The consequences? Oh, they're pretty significant. First off, you get poor-quality sleep, which leads to a *whole* list of issues. We're talking about impaired cognitive function (so you forget where you put your keys and wonder why you walked into the kitchen), mood instability (you're either crying over spilled milk or laughing like a maniac at a cat video), and a weakened immune system (which means you're more likely to catch that cold that's going around).

Health Risks of Disruption

But wait—there's more! Messing with your circadian rhythm doesn't just make you cranky and forgetful. Oh no, it can also increase your risk of some seriously unpleasant health issues. The longer you disrupt your sleep cycle, the higher the likelihood of developing metabolic disorders like obesity or diabetes. Why? Because irregular sleep wreaks havoc on your hormones, including those pesky ones like *ghrelin* (the hunger hormone) and *leptin* (the "I'm full" hormone), leading you to overeat and crave all the sugary snacks your heart desires.

And, as if that weren't enough, circadian misalignment can also contribute to cardiovascular diseases and even cancer. Yep, that's right—your poor sleep habits can increase your risk of some serious health conditions. Think of it like this: every time you stay up late or ignore your internal clock, you're potentially setting the stage for a bigger health issue down the road.

It's also worth noting that disrupted circadian rhythms can contribute to *inflammation*. And guess what? Chronic inflammation is linked to a whole host of diseases, from autoimmune disorders to heart disease. It's like your body's version of a fire that just won't go out, affecting everything from your joints to your arteries.

Hormonal Havoc

One of the major players in this whole disruption game is your hormones. Sleep disruption throws off the delicate balance of your hormone production. When you don't get enough sleep, your body releases higher levels of stress hormones, like *cortisol*, which can mess with everything from your blood sugar to your mood. Imagine trying to function with your hormones all out of whack— it's like trying to have a calm, productive day while your body's throwing a temper tantrum.

Circadian Rhythm and Modern Life: The Challenge of Synchronizing with Nature

In a world dominated by technology, long work hours, and never-ending Netflix binges, syncing your circadian rhythm with nature feels a little like trying to do yoga on a tightrope. But it's not impossible. Let's talk about the challenges we face, and how you can stop your internal clock from staging a revolt.

The Impact of Technology on Sleep

Let's get real—our smartphones, laptops, and TVs have become our bedtime buddies. It's like our internal clock has gone from "time for bed" to "let's scroll through Instagram one more time!" But that little blue light glowing from your screen? It's not helping you achieve your beauty sleep goals. In fact, it's messing with your internal clock, and not in a good way.

Blue light, the kind emitted from screens, is like that annoying friend who keeps talking during the movie: it totally interrupts your vibe. Here's the deal: when you expose yourself to blue light, your body gets confused. It thinks it's still daytime, and the production of *melatonin* — that sleep hormone your body so kindly produces to lull you into dreamland — gets suppressed. Instead of winding down, your body is wide awake, ready to take on the world at midnight.

If you're the type who likes to check emails right before bed (guilty as charged), you might be wondering why you're lying there staring at the ceiling, wondering why sleep feels like an urban myth. The culprit? That little blue glow. To help your circadian rhythm stay intact, try to avoid bright screens at least an hour before bed.

Practical Tips for Limiting Screen Time in the Evening

OK, I know, *not checking Instagram* is a big ask in the digital age, but trust me — your circadian rhythm will thank you. Here are some ways to keep your phone from becoming your bedtime enemy:

1. Use Night Mode: If you absolutely must stare at your phone, switch it to night mode. It reduces blue light, and while it's not a magic cure, it helps a little.
2. Set a "No-Screens" Zone: Try to make your bedroom a screen-free sanctuary. Use your bedroom for sleep and relaxation, not as a late-night work office or social media marathon center.

3. Switch to Paper Books: Old school, yes. But reading an actual book can help your mind relax, while also not emitting any blue light.

4. Blue Light Glasses: If you can't part with your phone, there are blue light-blocking glasses. They're like the armor for your eyes in the battle of the screens!

Shift Work and Jet Lag

You know who's really got it tough? Shift workers and frequent flyers. The constant switching between night shifts and day shifts can seriously mess with your circadian rhythm. It's like trying to get your internal clock to do the cha-cha, but it keeps tripping over its own feet. And don't even get me started on jet lag. Nothing says "you're messed up" like waking up at 3 a.m. and trying to pretend it's time for breakfast when you've just arrived at your destination.

So how do you fight the battle of the body clock when your schedule is all over the place? Well, here are a few tricks to help you manage shift work and jet lag.

1. Shift Work Survival: If you're stuck working odd hours, try to sync your sleep with the time you're supposed to be awake. If you're working nights, try to sleep in a dark, quiet room during the day (you might need blackout curtains and earplugs — become best friends with them).

2. Light Therapy: For shift workers and jet setters, exposure to the right light at the right time can be a game-changer. Get outside during daylight hours to reset your internal clock.

3. Meal Timing: Eating at the "wrong" time can confuse your body too. Try to adjust your meals to match your new schedule — if you're working nights, try eating your "breakfast" before your shift starts. It sounds weird, but it helps.

Syncing Your Circadian Rhythm for Better Health

Now that we've explored how technology, shift work, and jet lag throw a wrench into our circadian rhythm, let's talk about how to get your body back in sync with nature. Spoiler alert: It's not as complicated as it sounds, but it does require a little effort (and maybe fewer late-night Netflix binges).

Morning Light Exposure: Start Your Day Right

Here's a golden rule for a better day: Sunlight. Yes, that giant ball of fire in the sky that people forget about sometimes. The first thing you should do after waking up is get some natural light. Aim for 10 to 15 minutes of sunshine in the morning to kickstart your circadian rhythm. It's like a little wake-up call to your brain: "Hey, it's time to get up and be fabulous!"

Getting morning sunlight not only helps you feel more alert but also improves your mood. So, you can kill two birds with one stone: wake up feeling energized and happy. Bonus points if you combine this with a nice cup of coffee, but please, no coffee right after waking up. It's better to hydrate first.

Evening Habits: Wind Down, Don't Rev Up

When evening rolls around, it's time to start winding down, not gearing up for a second wind. Your body wants to know that bedtime is near, so here are some simple evening habits to help you signal to your body that it's time to sleep, not run a marathon:

1. Dim the Lights: Bright lights at night confuse your body into thinking it's still daytime. Start dimming the lights an hour or two before bed to help your body release melatonin and get into the sleep zone.
2. Red Light: Yes, you heard that right. Red light has less of an impact on your circadian rhythm and helps promote sleep. So, consider getting some red light bulbs for your bedroom.

3. Avoid Blue Light: As we discussed earlier, keep the screens away. You're not getting a good night's sleep with a phone in your hand.
4. Herbal Teas & Relaxation: Sip on some herbal teas (chamomile or valerian root are great) and practice relaxation techniques like deep breathing, meditation, or reading a book. These activities help ease your mind and body into sleep mode.

Regular Sleep Schedule: Consistency Is Key

You've probably heard it a million times: consistency is key. The same rule applies to your sleep schedule. Going to bed and waking up at the same time every day — even on weekends — will help your body lock in a rhythm. And no, hitting the snooze button repeatedly doesn't count as "getting in sync." Trust me, your body will thank you when it learns when to expect its regular rest.

You don't have to get up at 5 a.m. every day (unless you're into that), but sticking to a regular schedule will help improve the quality of your sleep. Plus, it'll make you feel less like a zombie.

The Impact of Sleep Duration on Health

Lastly, let's talk about the duration of sleep. Everyone is different, but getting at least 7 to 8 hours of quality sleep is non-negotiable. Think of it like charging your phone: If you only give it 3 hours, it's going to be dead by lunchtime. Your body needs time to rest, repair, and refresh.

The right amount of sleep is vital for brain function, mood regulation, and immune health. So, be kind to yourself. Your circadian rhythm is your best friend, and the more you align with it, the better your body will function.

How to Adjust Your Circadian Rhythm to Fit Your Lifestyle

Adaptation for Night Owls and Early Birds

Let's face it—some people are just wired to be night owls, while others greet the morning with the enthusiasm of a well-rested squirrel. If you're the former, the idea of waking up at 6 a.m. might sound about as appealing as a root canal, and if you're the latter, staying up past 9 p.m. might have you feeling like you're pushing the boundaries of human endurance. But what if your circadian rhythm doesn't match your work schedule or social life? Fear not! It is possible to adjust, and we've got tips to help make the transition painless.

For night owls trying to ease into earlier sleep habits, start slow. Don't expect your body to magically shift from staying up until 2 a.m. to being in bed by 10 p.m. (unless you're some sort of sleep wizard, in which case, teach me your ways). Instead, gradually move your bedtime earlier by 15–30 minutes each night. It's like convincing your body to go to bed a little earlier without feeling like it's being forced into a straightjacket.

On the flip side, if you're an early riser trying to stay up for late-night activities, try adjusting your routine in small increments. You can shift your bedtime later by 15–30 minutes each night until you're comfortably staying up later, but not at the expense of a grumpy morning. It's like training your body to stay up late without turning into a zombie the next day.

Balancing Social and Work Obligations

So you've got work deadlines to meet and friends who insist on late-night karaoke. What now? It's a delicate balancing act, like juggling flaming swords while blindfolded (metaphorically, of course). But all jokes aside, it's important to find a way to accommodate your social life and work obligations without completely sabotaging your circadian rhythm.

The key is consistency. If you've had a crazy late night with friends, try to get back on track the next night by sticking to your usual bedtime. Don't let one late night snowball into a whole week of bad sleep. Similarly, don't let work demands keep you up late every night—find ways to manage your workload to allow for proper rest. Think of it like meal prepping for sleep: plan ahead, and you'll be much less likely to skip the important stuff (like sleep).

Make sleep a priority, even when deadlines are looming or your social calendar is packed. Remember, not getting enough sleep will eventually catch up with you, and it'll be harder to catch up on rest than it is to catch up on Netflix shows. So, even if your boss or best friend is pleading for a late-night Zoom meeting or party, politely decline and tell them you're investing in your future well-being (and maybe you can send them a cute meme in the morning).

Future Research and Developments in Circadian Rhythm Science

Exploring the Role of Genetics

Turns out, your circadian rhythm might not just be about when you wake up and fall asleep—it could be written into your DNA. The fascinating field of chronobiology is exploring how our genetic makeup influences our sleep-wake cycles. It's like finding out that your body has a built-in timer that's genetically predetermined. Imagine that: your internal alarm clock could be uniquely yours, and it's possible that some people are just destined to be morning people while others are, unfortunately, stuck being night owls (no matter how many sleep apps they download).

This could eventually lead to personalized sleep therapies, where your genetic predispositions will help doctors create a tailored plan to optimize your sleep. You'll get advice that fits your personal circadian rhythm, so you'll no longer have to try to fit yourself into the "one-size-fits-all" sleep solution. So if your genetics say you're more of a night owl, don't feel guilty; embrace it!

The Promise of Circadian Medicine

But wait, there's more! Circadian rhythm science isn't just for sleep—there's growing evidence that it could be the key to treating chronic conditions. Imagine a future where doctors prescribe treatments that work *with* your circadian rhythm instead of against it. Instead of simply popping pills or trying generic treatments, you'd receive therapies timed to optimize your body's natural rhythms. If that doesn't sound like sci-fi turned reality, I don't know what does.

From improving sleep disorders to managing metabolic health, the future of circadian medicine is bright. And as we dive deeper into how the body's clock influences everything from digestion to brain function, we might see even more revolutionary treatments based on when we do things—like eating, exercising, and even taking medications—rather than just what we do.

Harnessing the Power of Your Internal Clock

So, here we are at the end of our circadian journey—your internal clock, or should I say *the VIP of your body's operations*, has had its time in the spotlight. And let's be honest, this isn't some boring timepiece that just ticks away in the corner. No, no, your circadian rhythm is like that one friend who always keeps things running on time, reminding you when to eat, sleep, and generally function like a human being. So, if you've been ignoring it all this time, it's high time you give it the credit it deserves.

By now, you should have a clear picture of why syncing with your body's natural rhythm is essential for everything from better sleep to higher productivity. It's not just about making sure you're awake when you should be or asleep when the world expects you to be. Oh no, it's about unlocking your superpowers — the ones that make you more energetic, more focused, and, let's face it, less likely to be that zombie at 3 p.m. trying to get through your workday. Your circadian rhythm is the backstage crew that makes your daily performance a success.

Here's the thing: You've got the power to take control of your own sleep habits. Yes, you! You don't need to let life's chaos dictate when you rest. We know, there are work deadlines, Netflix shows, and that one friend who always wants to meet up for a late-night chat about life. But what if, instead of battling your body's natural urges, you worked *with* them? By honoring your circadian rhythm — scheduling some morning sunlight, embracing your evening wind-down routine, and getting consistent sleep — you're giving yourself the gift of better energy, focus, and long-term health.

Imagine this: You wake up feeling refreshed, not grumpy, because your body's internal clock is in sync. You breeze through meetings without a caffeine IV drip, and your workouts actually feel, well, like workouts rather than something to just survive. And best of all, your mood? It's more like a breeze on a sunny day, instead of a storm cloud that follows you around.

Embracing the circadian rhythm isn't just about ticking off boxes on some sleep hygiene checklist. It's about understanding that your body has a natural flow, and when you respect that flow, you're in for a life filled with better sleep, a clearer mind, and enough energy to power through your day with a smile. No more feeling sluggish or like you need five cups of coffee just to get through the first hour of your workday.

In the long run, syncing with your circadian rhythm isn't a temporary fix. It's a transformation. It's like hitting the reset button on your health, turning you into the version of yourself that you're actually meant to be. So, the next time you're tempted to pull an all-nighter or push your bedtime back just to finish one more episode of your favorite show, remember that your body knows best. Trust it, and let it guide you toward a healthier, happier, and more productive life.

Now go ahead—start living in sync with your internal clock and watch how your health, mood, and energy transform. Who knew a little light, sleep, and routine could unlock so much? Time to thrive, my friend!

Detox and Fasting – The Ancient Art of Saying No to Food

For centuries, humans have practiced fasting and detoxification — sometimes by necessity, sometimes by tradition, and increasingly now, by choice. Ancient civilizations swore by the power of fasting for spiritual and physical renewal, while traditional medicine emphasized natural detoxification methods to cleanse the body of impurities. Today, science confirms what our ancestors instinctively knew: giving the body a break from constant digestion and exposure to toxins can trigger profound healing.

But let's clear something up — fasting and detox are *not* the same thing. While fasting is about pausing food intake to activate cellular repair, detox focuses on enhancing the body's natural elimination processes. Think of it this way: fasting is like hitting the reset button, while detox is the deep cleaning that follows. Together, they create a powerful synergy that can boost energy, improve digestion, and even sharpen mental clarity.

So, how exactly does fasting trigger detox? And why do some people feel *amazing* while others feel like they've been hit by a truck? More importantly, how can you do it *right* without falling for gimmicky "detox teas" or extreme fasting fads? Let's dive in.

> # DETOX SMOOTHIES
> *because your liver deserves a love letter in*
> # LIQUID FORM

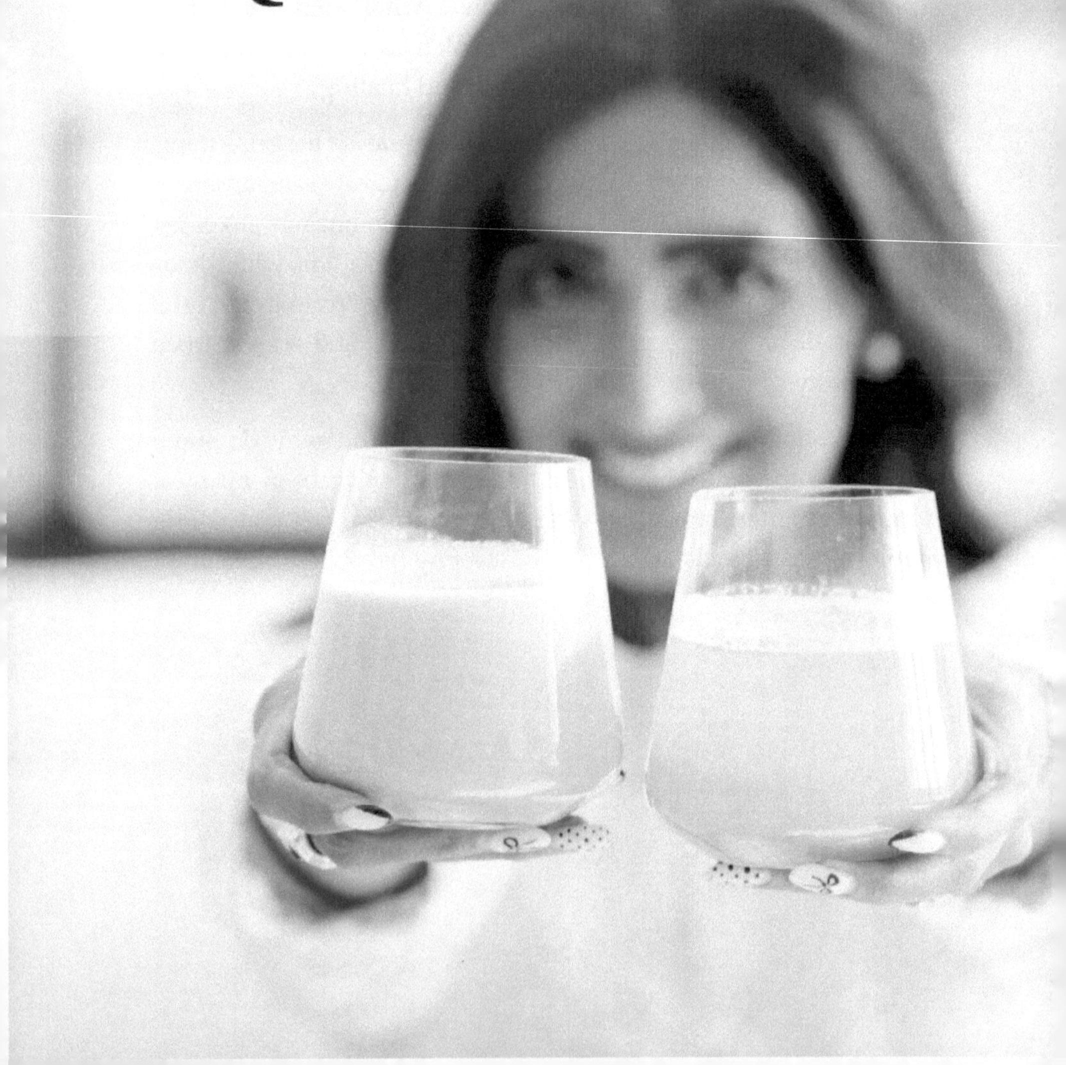

Understanding Detoxification: The Body's Hidden Superpower

Imagine your body as a high-performance machine, constantly running, processing, and filtering out waste. Now, just like any machine, it needs regular maintenance—this is where detoxification comes in. Contrary to what trendy detox diets might suggest, your body already has a sophisticated built-in detox system working 24/7.

What is Detox, Really?

Forget the hype around expensive juices and miracle cleanses—detoxification isn't about starving yourself or drinking questionable green concoctions. It's your body's natural way of eliminating toxins, balancing chemicals, and keeping everything running smoothly. Every day, you're exposed to toxins from food, air, water, and even stress. Your body, however, is built to handle them—if you give it the right tools.

Meet the Detox Dream Team: The Organs in Charge

Detoxification is not just a one-organ job—it's a full-body operation involving multiple systems working together to keep you healthy. Each organ plays a unique role in filtering toxins, breaking down waste, and ensuring harmful substances don't linger in your body. Here's a closer look at the key players in your body's natural detox system:

1. Liver: The Body's Primary Filter

The liver is often called the **master detoxifier**, and for good reason—it's your body's built-in purification system. Everything you eat, drink, and even absorb through your skin eventually passes through the liver for processing.

How It Works:

- The liver converts harmful substances (like alcohol, drugs, and environmental toxins) into less toxic compounds or water-soluble forms that can be excreted through urine or bile.
- It metabolizes fats, proteins, and carbohydrates while filtering out harmful substances from your bloodstream.
- It produces bile, which helps break down fats and flush out toxins via the digestive system.

Why It Matters:

If your liver is overburdened — due to excessive alcohol, processed foods, or environmental pollutants — it struggles to function efficiently. This can lead to toxin buildup, hormonal imbalances, and sluggish metabolism.

2. Kidneys: The Personal Filtration System

Your kidneys act like a high-efficiency filtration unit, ensuring your blood stays clean and balanced. Every day, they filter around 50 gallons of blood, removing excess fluids, waste, and toxins.

How They Work:

- The kidneys filter out waste products, toxins, and excess minerals from the blood, which are then eliminated through urine.
- They regulate fluid levels, ensuring the body stays properly hydrated and electrolyte levels remain balanced.
- They help maintain blood pressure and remove metabolic waste products like urea and creatinine.

Why They Matter:

Dehydration, excessive salt intake, and high levels of processed foods can strain the kidneys, making them work harder to remove toxins. Over time, this can lead to kidney stones, infections, and reduced detoxification efficiency.

3. Lymphatic System: The Unsung Hero

The lymphatic system is often overlooked in detox discussions, but it's essential in flushing out waste at the cellular level. Think of it as a garbage disposal network for your body.

How It Works:

- The lymphatic system consists of lymph nodes, vessels, and fluid that transport toxins, bacteria, and cellular waste out of the body.
- It works closely with the immune system to remove pathogens and support immune function.
- Unlike the circulatory system, which has the heart to pump blood, the lymphatic system relies on movement (exercise, massage, deep breathing) to circulate fluids and remove waste.

Why It Matters:

A sluggish lymphatic system can lead to toxin buildup, fluid retention, weakened immunity, and even skin issues like puffiness and acne. Movement, dry brushing, and staying hydrated help keep lymph flowing properly.

4. Gut: The Center of Digestion and Detox

Your gut is home to trillions of bacteria that play a vital role in breaking down food, absorbing nutrients, and eliminating waste.

When gut health is compromised, detoxification slows down, leading to bloating, sluggish digestion, and toxin reabsorption.

How It Works:

- The digestive tract eliminates toxins via bowel movements. A fiber-rich diet ensures waste is efficiently expelled.
- Beneficial gut bacteria help break down toxins, reducing their harmful effects before they enter the bloodstream.
- The gut lining acts as a barrier, preventing harmful substances from leaking into the bloodstream (a condition known as "leaky gut").

Why It Matters:

A poor diet, stress, and overuse of antibiotics can disrupt gut bacteria, leading to digestive issues, inflammation, and inefficient detoxification. Probiotics, fiber, and whole foods support gut health and toxin elimination.

5. Skin: The Largest Detox Organ

Your skin is more than just a protective barrier—it's also a **detox powerhouse** that expels toxins through sweat. If the liver and kidneys are overwhelmed, toxins may try to exit through the skin, leading to breakouts, rashes, and dullness.

How It Works:

- Sweat glands help flush out toxins like heavy metals and excess salt.
- The skin acts as a secondary route for detox when other organs are overburdened.
- A healthy skincare routine and proper hydration support the skin's detoxification process.

Why It Matters:

Excessive toxin buildup can show up as acne, dryness, or skin irritation. Regular exercise, hydration, and saunas help open up pores and release toxins effectively.

Detoxification isn't about extreme cleanses — it's about supporting your body's natural ability to process and remove waste. By keeping your liver, kidneys, lymphatic system, gut, and skin healthy, you're ensuring your detox team functions at its best. Simple habits like staying hydrated, eating whole foods, exercising, and managing stress can go a long way in optimizing your body's detox processes.

How to Support Your Detox System (Without Starving Yourself)

Detoxing isn't about extreme cleanses, juice fasts, or deprivation — it's about supporting your body's natural ability to remove waste and function optimally. Your body already has an incredible detox system (liver, kidneys, gut, lymphatic system, and skin), and all it needs is the right tools to work efficiently. Here's how you can help it, without resorting to drastic measures:

1. Hydration: Your Best Detoxifier

Water is one of the most powerful and natural detoxifiers available, playing a crucial role in supporting every detox organ by flushing out waste, transporting essential nutrients, and maintaining overall balance in the body. Proper hydration is essential for kidney function, as it helps filter out toxins and waste products like urea and excess sodium, preventing kidney stones and infections. It also plays a key role in lymphatic drainage, ensuring that fluids move efficiently to clear out toxins — without enough water, the lymphatic system can become sluggish, leading to bloating and toxin buildup. Additionally, water supports gut health by softening stool and preventing constipation, which is vital for the efficient elimination of waste and toxins. Hydration also benefits the skin, as well-hydrated skin is more effective at sweating out toxins, reducing breakouts, and promoting a natural glow.

To optimize hydration, it's important to drink at least **2-3 liters of water daily**, adjusting for activity levels and climate. Starting the day with **warm lemon water** can aid digestion and support liver function, while incorporating **coconut water** provides added electrolytes that enhance hydration. To maintain proper fluid balance, it's best to **limit dehydrating drinks** such as excessive coffee, alcohol, and sugary sodas, which can counteract the body's ability to retain and utilize water efficiently.

2. Clean Eating: Fuel Your Detox System

Your body detoxes more efficiently when it receives the right nutrients. Consuming highly processed foods, refined sugar, and trans fats can overburden the liver and slow down the detoxification process. In contrast, whole, nutrient-dense foods provide the essential vitamins, minerals, and antioxidants needed to support the body's natural cleansing functions. Leafy greens like spinach, kale, and cilantro are rich in chlorophyll, which helps neutralize toxins and aids liver function. Cruciferous vegetables such as broccoli, cauliflower, and Brussels sprouts contain compounds that activate liver detoxification pathways, making it easier for the body to process and eliminate harmful substances. Fiber-rich foods, including flaxseeds, chia seeds, and whole grains, play a crucial role in digestive health by promoting regular bowel movements, ensuring that toxins don't linger in the body. Additionally, vitamin C-rich fruits like citrus, berries, and papaya help boost the immune system and support liver function, while healthy fats from avocados, nuts, and olive oil reduce inflammation and assist in cellular detoxification.

To optimize your diet for detoxification, it's important to focus on whole, unprocessed foods rather than packaged options filled with preservatives and artificial chemicals. Increasing fiber intake can further aid digestion and facilitate waste elimination. Reducing sugar and alcohol consumption is also essential, as both can overwork the liver and contribute to toxin buildup. Additionally, incorporating protein-rich foods such as legumes, lean meats, and eggs helps support liver enzyme production, ensuring that detoxification pathways function efficiently. By making these mindful dietary choices, you can help your body cleanse itself naturally and maintain optimal health.

3. Herbal Teas: Nature's Detox Tonics

For centuries, herbal teas have been valued for their ability to aid digestion, cleanse the liver, and support kidney function. Incorporating these teas into your daily routine can be a gentle yet effective way to enhance the body's natural detoxification process. Dandelion tea is particularly beneficial for liver health, acting as a natural diuretic that helps flush out toxins through urine. Green tea, packed with antioxidants known as catechins, supports liver function while reducing oxidative stress caused by toxins and free radicals. For those struggling with sluggish digestion, ginger tea can be a game changer, as it stimulates circulation, aids digestion, and reduces inflammation. Meanwhile, peppermint tea is excellent for soothing digestive discomfort and relieving bloating, making it a great option after heavy meals. Turmeric tea, rich in curcumin, provides powerful anti-inflammatory benefits and further supports liver detoxification by encouraging the breakdown of harmful substances.

To incorporate herbal teas into your daily routine, aim for one to two cups per day as part of your hydration strategy. A warm cup of lemon-ginger tea in the morning can stimulate digestion and kickstart metabolism, while a refreshing cup of green tea in the afternoon provides an antioxidant boost and helps improve focus. Making herbal teas a daily habit not only supports detoxification but also promotes overall well-being, keeping your body balanced and energized.

4. Saunas & Sweat Sessions: Detox Through Your Skin

Sweating is one of the body's most effective ways to eliminate toxins, including heavy metals, alcohol, and environmental pollutants. When you don't sweat regularly, these toxins can accumulate in fat cells, leading to fatigue, skin problems, and a sluggish detox system. By opening up pores and flushing out impurities, sweating helps eliminate harmful substances such as lead, mercury, and arsenic. It also boosts circulation, ensuring that oxygen and nutrients reach vital organs while promoting a healthy immune response and reducing inflammation.

To maximize detox through sweating, consider incorporating saunas, exercise, hot baths, and dry brushing into your routine. A 15-20 minute infrared sauna session encourages deep sweating, helping remove toxins at a cellular level. Regular exercise, including cardio, strength training, and yoga, not only promotes sweating but also improves blood circulation and lymphatic drainage. Hot baths with Epsom salt further enhance detox by drawing out impurities and relaxing the muscles. Additionally, dry brushing, a gentle exfoliation technique, stimulates the lymphatic system and promotes toxin elimination through the skin. By making sweat-inducing activities a part of your lifestyle, you support your body's natural detoxification process while improving overall health and vitality.

5. Gut Health Focus: The Key to Efficient Detoxification

Your gut plays a central role in detoxification, acting as both a filter and a defense system. It processes waste, absorbs essential nutrients, and prevents harmful substances from re-entering your bloodstream. However, when your gut microbiome is imbalanced, toxins can accumulate, leading to bloating, brain fog, sluggish digestion, and even systemic inflammation. A healthy gut microbiome supports detox by ensuring that toxins are broken down and eliminated efficiently. Probiotics, or beneficial bacteria, help prevent the overgrowth of harmful microbes, while prebiotics (found in foods like garlic, onions, and bananas) serve as fuel for these good bacteria, keeping your digestive system in balance.

To optimize gut health for effective detox, include fermented foods like kimchi, yogurt, kefir, and sauerkraut in your diet, as they naturally support digestion and gut function. Fiber-rich foods such as legumes, whole grains, and vegetables promote regular bowel movements, preventing toxin buildup. Additionally, limiting processed foods, artificial additives, and preservatives helps reduce gut inflammation and prevents harmful substances from disrupting your microbiome. Staying properly hydrated is also crucial, as it supports digestion and ensures waste is flushed out rather than being reabsorbed into the bloodstream. By taking care of your gut, you enhance your body's natural detoxification process, leading to better digestion, improved energy levels, and overall well-being.

A Sustainable Approach to Detox

Detoxing isn't about starving yourself or following extreme juice cleanses—it's about supporting your body in the way it was designed to function. Your liver, kidneys, gut, and skin are constantly working to eliminate toxins, and the best thing you can do is give them the right tools to do their job efficiently. Hydration is key—something as simple as drinking enough water can make a huge difference in flushing out waste. Eating clean, whole foods nourishes your body with essential nutrients while reducing the toxic load from processed foods. Herbs and antioxidants give your liver an extra boost, helping it break down harmful substances more effectively. And let's not forget about movement—sweating through exercise or sauna sessions is a powerful way to release toxins and rejuvenate your system.

One of the most overlooked but crucial parts of detox is gut health—if your digestion isn't functioning properly, toxins can linger in your system instead of being eliminated. That's why adding probiotics, fiber, and fermented foods into your routine can make all the difference. The best part? You don't have to overhaul your life or suffer through restrictive detox programs. Small, sustainable habits add up, and when you prioritize balance over extremes, you'll start feeling lighter, more energized, and truly refreshed. Detoxing should never feel like a punishment—it should feel like self-care.

Understanding Fasting: A Natural Detox Mechanism

Fasting is more than just skipping meals—it's a strategic break from food that allows your body to repair, reset, and eliminate toxins. When done correctly, fasting enhances cellular function, improves metabolism, and supports deep detoxification without depriving your body of essential nutrients.

Fasting is an ancient practice that has been used for spiritual, medical, and health reasons across cultures. While many people associate fasting with simply not eating, different types of fasting have unique effects on the body, particularly when it comes to detoxification and cellular repair. Below, we'll explore the three main types of fasting—**dry fasting, water fasting, and intermittent fasting**—and how each supports overall well-being.

1. Dry Fasting: The Most Intense Detox

Dry fasting is the most extreme form of fasting, where you completely abstain from both food and water for a certain period.

Unlike other fasting methods that allow hydration, dry fasting forces the body to rely entirely on internal resources to sustain energy and maintain hydration. When deprived of external water sources, the body adapts by extracting moisture from fat cells and metabolizing it into metabolic water. This internally generated water is exceptionally pure, aiding in the removal of deeply stored toxins and impurities. Additionally, dry fasting triggers a powerful biological process called autophagy, where the body identifies and breaks down old, damaged, or malfunctioning cells, recycling them for energy. This deep cellular renewal helps eliminate waste far more effectively than other fasting methods.

One of the most significant benefits of dry fasting is its ability to boost the immune system. Since bacteria, viruses, and other pathogens thrive in hydrated environments, temporary dehydration creates unfavorable conditions for these harmful organisms, reducing their survival rate. This makes dry fasting a powerful tool for detoxification, as it not only cleanses the body at a cellular level but also strengthens its natural defense mechanisms. Moreover, by eliminating external food and water intake, the body's energy is redirected toward repair and regeneration, rather than digestion. This results in reduced inflammation, accelerated fat breakdown, and the elimination of toxins stored within fat cells.

Despite its incredible benefits, dry fasting should be approached with caution. Due to the intensity of the process, beginners should limit their fasting duration to 12–24 hours and gradually increase their tolerance. It is not suitable for individuals with kidney issues, dehydration risks, or chronic health conditions, as the absence of water can put additional strain on the body. After completing a dry fast, it is crucial to rehydrate properly and consume nutrient-dense foods to replenish lost minerals and electrolytes. When done mindfully and in moderation, dry fasting serves as a powerful detoxification practice, promoting cellular regeneration, immune resilience, and overall health.

2. Water Fasting: Cellular Renewal & Deep Detox

Water fasting is a method of fasting where an individual consumes only water for a set period, completely avoiding all solid foods, juices, or calorie-containing beverages. Unlike dry fasting, which eliminates both food and water, water fasting is a gentler yet highly effective approach to detoxification and cellular repair. It allows the body to reset and heal while still maintaining hydration. During water fasting, digestion, which typically consumes a significant amount of energy, is put on hold. This enables the body to redirect its energy toward internal processes such as deep cellular repair, detoxification, and metabolic optimization. One of the key mechanisms activated during water fasting is ketosis, where the body shifts from using glucose (carbohydrates) as its primary fuel source to burning stored fat for energy. Since toxins are often stored in fat cells, this breakdown process facilitates their release and elimination, further enhancing the body's natural detox pathways. Additionally, water fasting triggers autophagy, a cellular cleansing process in which damaged or dysfunctional cells are broken down and recycled. This not only supports detoxification but also reduces inflammation, improves overall cell function, and enhances longevity.

The detoxification benefits of water fasting are substantial. The liver and kidneys, the body's primary detox organs, function more efficiently, flushing out metabolic waste and accumulated toxins. The digestive system also gets a much-needed reset, reducing bloating and gut inflammation while improving nutrient absorption once eating resumes. Moreover, as the body burns fat for fuel, it naturally sheds excess weight while simultaneously eliminating stored toxins. Another significant benefit of water fasting is its impact on brain function. The process increases levels of brain-derived neurotrophic factor (BDNF), a protein that supports brain health, enhances cognitive function, and promotes mental clarity. Many individuals report improved focus, heightened awareness, and emotional stability during water fasting due to reduced inflammation and better neuronal communication.

For those new to water fasting, it is crucial to begin gradually. Beginners should start with 12 to 24-hour fasts before progressing to longer durations such as 48 or 72 hours. Staying hydrated is essential, with a recommended intake of 2–3 liters of water per day to support kidney function and toxin elimination. It is also important to break the fast gently to avoid digestive distress. Light, nutrient-dense foods such as bone broth, fresh fruits, and steamed vegetables should be reintroduced slowly to allow the digestive system to ease back into processing food. Proper refeeding ensures that the body retains the benefits of fasting while minimizing any discomfort. With the right approach, water fasting can be a powerful tool for cellular renewal, detoxification, and overall well-being.

3. Intermittent Fasting (IF): A Sustainable Detox Approach

Intermittent fasting (IF) is one of the most accessible and sustainable forms of fasting, allowing individuals to experience the benefits of fasting without extreme deprivation. Unlike prolonged fasting methods, IF involves cycling between periods of eating and fasting either daily or weekly. This approach helps the body transition between a fed and fasting state, improving metabolic flexibility and overall health. During fasting periods, the digestive system gets a much-needed break, reducing gut inflammation and promoting detoxification. Additionally, the body begins to burn stored fat for energy, gradually releasing toxins that accumulate in fat cells. One of the key advantages of IF is its ability to stimulate autophagy, a cellular repair process where the body removes damaged cells and regenerates new, healthy ones. This natural cleansing mechanism supports longevity, enhances energy levels, and improves overall well-being.

There are several popular IF methods that cater to different lifestyles and health goals. The 16:8 method involves fasting for 16 hours and consuming meals within an 8-hour window, such as eating between 12 PM and 8 PM while fasting from 8 PM to 12 PM the next day. This is one of the easiest and most widely practiced IF techniques. The 5:2 method follows a different pattern, where individuals eat normally for five days and restrict calorie intake to 500–600 calories on two non-consecutive days, such as Monday and Thursday. Another approach is alternate-day fasting, where people eat normally one day and then consume very low calories or only water the next day. Each of these methods allows the body to enter a fasting state long enough to trigger detoxification, fat burning, and cellular repair without feeling overly restrictive.

The detoxification benefits of IF are extensive. It encourages gradual and natural toxin removal without the extreme measures of prolonged fasting. Since fasting reduces gut inflammation and allows the digestive tract to heal, it significantly improves digestion and gut health. IF also helps regulate hormonal balance, particularly insulin and growth hormone levels, leading to better metabolism, increased fat burning, and sustained energy levels. Another critical advantage is its ability to reduce oxidative stress, which lowers the risk of chronic diseases and supports overall longevity.

To maximize the benefits of IF, it is essential to follow best practices. Choosing a fasting method that aligns with one's lifestyle and health needs ensures long-term sustainability. During eating windows, focusing on nutrient-dense meals, including whole foods rich in fiber, protein, and healthy fats, is crucial for maintaining energy and supporting detoxification. Staying hydrated is equally important—drinking plenty of water, herbal teas, and electrolyte-rich beverages prevents dehydration and enhances the body's natural cleansing processes. By incorporating intermittent fasting into daily life with a balanced approach, individuals can experience improved digestion, enhanced detoxification, and sustained well-being without the need for extreme dietary restrictions.

Which Fasting Method is Right for You?

Each fasting method offers unique benefits, making it important to choose one that aligns with your health goals and lifestyle. Dry fasting, the most intense form, triggers deep cellular repair and detoxification by eliminating damaged cells through autophagy. However, due to its intensity, it should only be done for short periods and with caution. Water fasting, on the other hand, provides a complete digestive reset, allowing the liver and kidneys to efficiently eliminate toxins while enhancing fat breakdown, where toxins are often stored. For those seeking a sustainable approach to detox and metabolism balance, intermittent fasting (IF) is ideal. IF cycles between periods of eating and fasting, with popular methods like 16:8 (fasting for 16 hours and eating within an 8-hour window) or 5:2 (eating normally for five days and restricting calories for two).

IF not only supports detoxification but also reduces inflammation, improves gut health, and stabilizes blood sugar levels. Regardless of the method chosen, it's crucial to listen to your body and adjust accordingly. Fasting, when done mindfully, isn't just about detox — it's a long-term lifestyle practice that enhances both physical and mental well-being, promoting sustained energy, better digestion, and overall vitality.

How Fasting Triggers Detoxification:

When you fast, your body shifts into a repair and renewal mode. Autophagy, a process where your body recycles damaged cells and removes toxins, is activated during fasting. Additionally, fasting allows the gut to heal, reducing bloating, improving digestion, and preventing harmful substances from re-entering your bloodstream. As your body burns stored fat for energy, it also releases and eliminates stored toxins, making fasting a natural way to support deep detoxification.

Fasting, when done mindfully and in alignment with your body's needs, can be a powerful tool for resetting your health and supporting long-term wellness. The key is to approach it with balance, ensuring you stay hydrated and nourish your body during eating windows.

The Role of Gut Health in Detox & Fasting: Your Inner Ecosystem

Ever wondered why some people can eat a bowl of raw veggies or a plate of lentils without any discomfort, while others feel bloated and sluggish? The answer lies in gut health—your body's internal ecosystem that plays a crucial role in digestion, detoxification, and overall well-being. Think of your gut as a bustling city, filled with trillions of bacteria working behind the scenes to break down food, absorb nutrients, and eliminate toxins. When this microbial balance is off, detoxing and fasting can feel more like a struggle than a reset. But with the right approach, you can turn your gut into a thriving powerhouse for better health.

Why Some People Struggle With Certain Foods

If eating fiber-rich foods like raw vegetables, legumes, or whole grains leaves you feeling bloated or uncomfortable, your gut bacteria—or lack thereof—could be the culprit. These foods require specific microbes to break them down and ferment fiber into short-chain fatty acids (SCFAs), which reduce inflammation and support detoxification. When those microbes are missing, fiber can sit in the gut, causing gas and discomfort. Instead of avoiding these foods, the goal should be to strengthen your gut so it can process them efficiently.

How to Improve Gut Health for Better Detox & Fasting

A well-balanced gut doesn't just help with digestion—it enhances detoxification, supports liver function, and even makes fasting easier. Here's how you can nourish your gut to get the most out of your detox and fasting routine:

1. Prebiotics & Probiotics: The Dynamic Duo of Gut Health

Your gut bacteria are like a garden—prebiotics act as fertilizer, while probiotics are the beneficial plants that keep the soil rich.

- **Prebiotics** are fibers that feed good bacteria, helping them thrive. Foods like garlic, onions, leeks, asparagus, bananas, and oats are excellent sources.
- **Probiotics** are live bacteria that help balance your gut microbiome. You'll find them in yogurt, kefir, kimchi, sauerkraut, miso, and kombucha. If your diet lacks fermented foods, high-quality probiotic supplements can give your gut the boost it needs.

2. Fermented Foods: Nature's Gut Healers

Fermented foods are like the superheroes of digestion, packed with probiotics and enzymes that make food easier to process.

- **Yogurt**: Rich in gut-friendly bacteria like Lactobacillus and Bifidobacteria, helping digestion and boosting immunity.
- **Kimchi & Sauerkraut**: Fermented cabbage powerhouses that improve gut flora and digestion.
- **Kombucha**: A fizzy, probiotic-rich tea that supports gut and liver health.
- **Miso & Tempeh**: Fermented soy products that enhance microbial diversity.

3. Gradual Dietary Shifts for a Resilient Gut

If your gut isn't used to fiber-rich or fermented foods, jumping in too fast can lead to bloating. Instead, ease into a gut-friendly diet:

- Start with small amounts of fiber and fermented foods, gradually increasing intake.
- Eat a variety of whole foods to promote bacterial diversity.
- Stay hydrated to support digestion and toxin elimination.
- Cut back on processed foods and sugar, which disrupt gut bacteria.

By nurturing your gut, detoxing and fasting become effortless, allowing your body to naturally reset, absorb nutrients efficiently, and eliminate toxins with ease. A thriving gut isn't just the key to better digestion—it's the foundation of a healthier, more energized life.

Common Mistakes & How to Avoid Them: A Smarter Approach to Detox & Fasting

Detoxing and fasting can be powerful tools for resetting your body, improving digestion, and enhancing overall health. However, when done incorrectly, they can backfire, leaving you feeling exhausted, deprived, and even harming your metabolism. Many people make common mistakes when attempting to detox or fast, often believing that "more is better" when, in reality, balance is key. Let's break down the most common pitfalls and how you can avoid them.

1. Overdoing Detox: Why Extreme Cleanses Fail

The idea of detoxing has been commercialized into juice cleanses, tea detoxes, and extreme diet plans that promise rapid results. While the body does need support in eliminating toxins, extreme detox methods often do more harm than good.

Why it's a mistake:

- Most extreme cleanses severely restrict calories and essential nutrients, which can slow metabolism and make you feel weak.
- Many detox programs eliminate proteins and healthy fats, both of which are crucial for liver function and cell repair.
- Relying on liquid-only cleanses for an extended period can lead to muscle loss, blood sugar imbalances, and increased cravings.

How to avoid it:

- Instead of extreme detoxes, focus on **sustainable** methods like increasing whole foods, drinking plenty of water, and reducing processed foods.
- Support your body with **natural detoxifiers** such as leafy greens, lemon water, turmeric, and fiber-rich foods that help eliminate toxins through digestion.
- Remember, **your liver, kidneys, and gut are naturally designed to detox**—they just need the right nutrients to function optimally.

2. Fasting Too Aggressively: How to Ease Into Fasting Safely

Fasting has many benefits, including improved metabolism, autophagy (cellular repair), and reduced inflammation. However, jumping into long fasting periods too quickly can shock the body and lead to dizziness, fatigue, and nutrient deficiencies.

Why it's a mistake:

- **Going from eating all day to extreme fasting (24-48 hours) too quickly** can stress the body, leading to headaches, low energy, and irritability.

- Not consuming **enough nutrients during eating windows** can cause muscle loss and slow down metabolism.
- Ignoring **electrolytes and hydration** can result in dizziness and dehydration.

How to avoid it:
- Start **gradually** by practicing intermittent fasting (such as the 12:12 or 16:8 method) before attempting longer fasts.
- **Prioritize whole, nutrient-dense foods** during your eating window, including healthy fats, proteins, and fiber to keep energy levels stable.
- Stay **hydrated** and include mineral-rich fluids like herbal teas, lemon water, and bone broth to support your system.

3. Not Prioritizing Gut Health Before Detox & Fasting

Your gut plays a **major role in detoxification** by breaking down food, absorbing nutrients, and eliminating waste. If your gut isn't functioning well, detoxing or fasting can lead to digestive discomfort, bloating, and nutrient deficiencies.

Why it's a mistake:
- A weak gut microbiome struggles to digest fiber, leading to bloating when consuming raw veggies or pulses.
- Detoxing without gut health support can lead to **constipation**, preventing toxins from being efficiently removed.
- Fasting without gut-friendly foods can cause imbalances in gut bacteria, weakening digestion in the long run.

How to avoid it:

- **Support your gut with prebiotics and probiotics** before starting a detox or fast. Foods like yogurt, kimchi, kefir, and sauerkraut help nourish gut bacteria.
- Increase **fiber intake gradually** to avoid digestive distress — start with cooked veggies before moving to raw.
- Stay **hydrated and include digestive-friendly teas**, like ginger and peppermint, to soothe the gut.

A Balanced Approach to Detox & Fasting

Detoxing and fasting aren't about depriving yourself — they're about working with your body, not against it. The goal isn't to suffer through extreme cleanses or push your limits, but to nourish your system in a way that supports natural detoxification. True wellness comes from hydration, whole foods, and antioxidants that help your body function at its best.

Fasting should feel like a reset, not a punishment — when done gradually and mindfully, it boosts energy, enhances metabolism, and gives your digestive system a well-deserved break. But the real game-changer? Gut health. Without a strong, balanced gut, your body struggles to absorb nutrients and eliminate toxins efficiently. Instead of searching for quick fixes, focus on long-term habits that make you feel good from the inside out.

When you approach detoxing and fasting as sustainable lifestyle choices rather than short-term challenges, you'll feel more energized, refreshed, and in tune with what your body truly needs.

Gut: The Unsung Hero of Your Health

I was just a child, maybe five years old, when I first began facing digestive issues. Constipation, bloating, and stomach discomfort became my constant companions as I grew older. Despite being part of a highly athletic family, where nutrition was considered sacred and "ghar ka khana" was the cure for everything, my body seemed to rebel against what was considered the ultimate healthy diet. Mornings began early, often at 4:35 AM, with intense sports like basketball and track running, yet my digestive struggles persisted.

Growing up, I followed the typical Indian stereotype of healthy eating—rotis, vegetables, milk, and protein. But despite my athleticism and disciplined routine, my gut wasn't cooperating. Visits to numerous doctors and hospitals provided little relief. I was prescribed every remedy and treatment under the sun, but nothing seemed to work. I continued to push through, living with these issues, but things took a turn for the worse after I gave birth to my daughter. No matter where I went, the advice was always the same: "*Eat more rotis rolled up with ghee and sugar, more vegetables, and more milk for protein.*"

I tried everything—from low-calorie diets to every fad that promised a quick fix. While I did lose weight after pregnancy, thanks to my age and metabolism, I constantly struggled with a bloated stomach and low energy levels. The weight loss wasn't due to prescribed remedies or dietary recommendations—it was the result of countless hours spent in the gym. Frustrated and drained by the endless cycle of medications and diets, I finally decided to take matters into my own hands. I began researching gut health, and that's when I had my breakthrough. What if gluten and dairy were the real culprits? What if my body had been reacting to them all along? So, I eliminated them from my diet—and to my surprise, the changes were nothing short of remarkable.

This realization opened a new chapter in my life—not only a journey to healing my gut but also a deeper understanding of nutrition and lifestyle. It's what ultimately led me to explore the fascinating world of gut health, and it's what I'll share with you in this chapter. Because sometimes, the road to feeling better is not about following conventional wisdom but about truly listening to your body and learning what works for you.

If your body were a high-tech factory, your gut would be the control center—handling digestion, immune responses, and even influencing your mood. Yet, we tend to take it for granted until something goes wrong. You know the drill—one bad meal, and suddenly, your gut reminds you who's really in charge.

But the gut is more than just a food-processing unit. Inside your digestive system lives an entire universe of bacteria, fungi, and other microscopic creatures—your gut microbiome—which plays a crucial role in keeping you healthy. Some call it the "second brain," and honestly, considering how much it affects your mood and decisions (like making you crave junk food at 2 AM), they might be onto something.

The gut microbiome consists of trillions of bacteria, both good and bad. When this delicate balance is disturbed—due to poor diet, stress, antibiotics, or lack of sleep—your overall health takes a hit. Symptoms like bloating, constipation, skin breakouts, fatigue, and even anxiety or depression can often be traced back to an unhappy gut.

For years, I ignored these signs, believing that pushing through discomfort was just a part of life. But as I delved deeper into gut health, I realized that healing doesn't come from merely treating symptoms — it requires addressing the root cause.

One of the first things I changed was my diet. I swapped out gluten-heavy foods for whole, fiber-rich alternatives and removed dairy, replacing it with plant-based options. I introduced fermented foods like kimchi and homemade yogurt, which are packed with probiotics that help restore gut flora. Hydration became a priority, with coconut water and herbal teas replacing sugary drinks. I also incorporated mindful eating habits — chewing slowly, avoiding overeating, and giving my digestive system the care it deserved.

But food wasn't the only piece of the puzzle. Stress plays a massive role in gut health. The gut and brain are connected through the gut-brain axis, meaning that high stress levels can disrupt digestion, trigger inflammation, and lead to issues like IBS. I started practicing meditation and deep breathing, and I noticed a shift in my overall well-being. Movement also became intentional — not just high-intensity workouts but gentle activities like yoga and walking, which promote gut motility and reduce stress.

Slowly but surely, my gut began to heal. The bloating reduced, my energy levels improved, and for the first time in years, I felt truly in tune with my body. This transformation wasn't about following a strict diet or obsessing over food rules — it was about understanding my body's needs and responding accordingly.

The more I learned, the more I realized how many people struggle with similar issues without realizing the root cause. Digestive problems, skin conditions, hormonal imbalances — so many of these can be traced back to the gut. Yet, we often overlook it, treating only the symptoms rather than addressing the underlying issue.

Healing your gut isn't a one-size-fits-all approach. What worked for me might not work for you, and that's okay. The key is to start small—listen to your body, identify trigger foods, and make gradual changes. Incorporate whole, unprocessed foods, stay hydrated, manage stress, and most importantly, be patient with yourself.

Your gut does more than digest food; it influences your immune system, mental health, and overall vitality. If there's one thing I've learned, it's that gut health isn't just about avoiding discomfort—it's about thriving. And when you take the time to nourish and care for your gut, it rewards you with energy, balance, and a renewed sense of well-being.

So, if you're struggling with digestion, feeling constantly bloated, or dealing with unexplained fatigue, start by looking inward—literally. Your gut might just be trying to tell you something. Are you ready to listen?

The Gut: More Than Just Digestion

Your gut, or gastrointestinal (GI) tract, is a 27-foot-long superhighway running from your mouth to your... well, you know where. It's responsible for breaking down food, absorbing nutrients, and eliminating waste. But digestion is just the tip of the iceberg.

1. The Gut Microbiome

Inside your intestines live trillions of bacteria, viruses, and fungi—collectively called the gut microbiome. These tiny tenants aren't just passive residents; they actively influence your digestion, metabolism, immune system, and even mental health.

The Role of Good Bacteria

Good bacteria are essential for maintaining a well-functioning digestive system. They help break down complex carbohydrates, produce short-chain fatty acids, and synthesize essential vitamins such as:

- **Vitamin B12:** Crucial for red blood cell formation, neurological function, and DNA synthesis.
- **Vitamin K:** Plays a key role in blood clotting and bone health.
- **Biotin (Vitamin B7):** Supports metabolism and promotes healthy hair, skin, and nails.
- **Folic Acid (Vitamin B9):** Essential for cell growth and development, particularly during pregnancy.
- **Thiamine (Vitamin B1):** Helps convert food into energy and supports nerve function.

In addition to these vitamins, beneficial bacteria also produce neurotransmitters like serotonin and dopamine, which play a role in regulating mood and emotional well-being. In fact, nearly 90% of serotonin is produced in the gut, further proving its link to mental health.

The Dangers of Bad Bacteria

While good bacteria work tirelessly to support your health, bad bacteria can wreak havoc when left unchecked. An overgrowth of harmful microbes can lead to:

- **Chronic Inflammation:** This is a root cause of many diseases, including arthritis, heart disease, and autoimmune conditions.
- **Gastrointestinal Disorders:** Conditions like irritable bowel syndrome (IBS), small intestinal bacterial overgrowth (SIBO), and acid reflux are often linked to an imbalance in gut bacteria.
- **Metabolic Issues:** Research suggests that gut dysbiosis (an imbalance of gut bacteria) can contribute to obesity, insulin resistance, and type 2 diabetes.

- **Weakened Immunity:** Since about 70% of the immune system resides in the gut, an unhealthy microbiome can lead to frequent infections and slower recovery from illnesses.

A balanced microbiome is key to a happy gut, but factors like poor diet, stress, antibiotics, lack of sleep, and an unhealthy lifestyle can throw it off balance, leading to all sorts of health problems. That's why taking care of your gut health is not just about digestion—it's about overall well-being.

2. Your Gut and the Brain: The Weird Connection

Ever had a "gut feeling" about something? Or felt butterflies in your stomach before an important event? That's not just a figure of speech—your gut and brain are in constant communication, woven together through the intricate gut-brain axis. This connection is so profound that what happens in your gut doesn't just stay there—it ripples through your entire emotional state, shaping how you feel, think, and even respond to the world around you.

Have you ever felt a pit in your stomach during heartbreak? Or lost your appetite when overwhelmed with anxiety? That's your gut reacting to your emotions. But what if I told you that the reverse is also true—your emotions react to your gut? The trillions of bacteria residing in your digestive system don't just process food; they produce neurotransmitters like serotonin (the "happiness hormone"), dopamine (the "pleasure and motivation hormone"), and GABA (which helps calm your nervous system).

In fact, nearly 90% of your body's serotonin isn't made in your brain—it's made in your gut. That means an unhealthy gut doesn't just lead to bloating or indigestion; it can lead to persistent mood swings, anxiety, irritability, and even depression. You may find yourself feeling on edge for no reason, experiencing brain fog that won't lift, or struggling to find motivation—even when everything in your life seems fine. It's as if your gut is carrying an emotional weight you don't fully understand.

And then there are the cravings — those insatiable urges for sugar, processed carbs, or junk food that hit hardest when you're stressed or feeling low. Ever wondered why? It's not just emotional eating — it's your gut bacteria calling the shots. When harmful bacteria take over, they hijack your cravings, demanding the very foods that keep them alive. The more sugar and processed food you consume, the more these bad microbes thrive, creating a vicious cycle that keeps you trapped in patterns of exhaustion, mood crashes, and emotional instability.

But here's the thing — your gut can also be your greatest ally in healing. When nourished with the right foods, lifestyle habits, and self-care, it has the power to transform your mental and emotional state. A balanced gut doesn't just improve digestion; it lifts brain fog, stabilizes mood, and even enhances resilience against stress.

So, if you've been feeling down lately, struggling with unexplained anxiety, or simply not feeling like yourself—it might not be "all in your head." It could be in your gut. And the good news? You have the power to change it.

3. The Immune System: Gut's Role in Keeping You Safe

Have you ever wondered why some people fall sick at the slightest change in weather while others rarely catch a cold? The answer might not just lie in their exposure to germs but in something much deeper — hidden in the very core of their bodies. A whopping 70% of your immune system is located in your gut! That's right — your digestive system is not just about breaking down food; it's a frontline defense mechanism, determining how well your body can fight infections, respond to allergens, and maintain overall health.

A Story of Immunity: A Battle Within Picture this: Every time you eat, your gut is like a bustling city, filled with microscopic inhabitants — bacteria, fungi, and other microorganisms — all working together (or against each other) to determine the fate of your health. In this city, the good bacteria act as security forces, training your immune cells to recognize real threats. They teach your body to differentiate between a harmless peanut and a dangerous virus, between friendly pollen and an actual infection.

But what happens when the balance shifts? When harmful bacteria take over, your immune system goes into overdrive, attacking everything in sight—even your own body. This overreaction leads to allergies, autoimmune disorders, and chronic inflammation. The gut, once your greatest protector, becomes a source of constant internal battles.

- **Gut and the Body:** Your gut isn't just connected to digestion; it influences nearly every organ system in your body. It communicates with your brain through the gut-brain axis, regulates metabolism, impacts heart health, and even plays a role in skin conditions like acne and eczema. An imbalanced gut can cause issues far beyond bloating or indigestion—it can lead to hormonal imbalances, unexplained fatigue, and chronic inflammation.

- **Toxins:** Every day, we're exposed to environmental toxins—from pesticides in our food to chemicals in skincare products. But did you know that your gut plays a crucial role in detoxification? A healthy gut efficiently processes and eliminates toxins, preventing them from entering your bloodstream. However, when your gut is compromised, these toxins seep into your body, triggering systemic inflammation, fatigue, and even brain fog. Supporting your gut with whole foods, fiber, and probiotics can help it do its job effectively.

- **Inflammation:** Inflammation is your body's natural response to injury or infection, but when it becomes chronic, it can lead to severe health problems. An imbalanced gut can cause systemic inflammation, which has been linked to conditions like arthritis, heart disease, and even Alzheimer's. If you're constantly feeling tired, experiencing joint pain, or struggling with digestive discomfort, it could be a sign of underlying inflammation rooted in your gut health.

- **Metabolism and the Gut:** Ever wondered why some people can eat anything and never gain weight while others struggle despite their best efforts? Your gut bacteria play a massive role in metabolism. They influence how efficiently you break down food, store fat, and even regulate hunger hormones. An unhealthy gut can lead to sluggish metabolism, increased fat storage, and uncontrollable cravings. Simply put, a well-balanced gut can help you manage your weight more effectively.

- **Skin Health:** Acne, eczema, psoriasis—these aren't just surface-level problems; they often start deep in your gut. When harmful bacteria take over, they release toxins that trigger skin inflammation, leading to persistent breakouts and other skin issues. Healing your skin isn't just about applying the right creams; it's about nourishing your gut with the right foods, hydration, and stress management.

- **Gastric Issues:** In many households, gastric issues like acidity, bloating, and constipation are considered "normal." Taking antacids, laxatives, or Eno has become a post-25 ritual, with people fearing the discomfort of skipping their daily dose. The mindset of tolerating digestive distress, rather than addressing the root cause, leads to dependency on quick fixes. But here's the truth—gut problems are not normal. They're a sign that your body is calling for help. Ignoring them now may lead to more severe issues down the line, from chronic inflammation to autoimmune conditions.

Breaking the Cycle: If you've been struggling with poor digestion, unexplained weight gain, skin issues, or constant fatigue, it's time to look inward—at your gut. Instead of reaching for another pill, consider:

- Reducing processed foods and refined sugars
- Eating a fiber-rich, whole-food diet
- Incorporating probiotic and prebiotic-rich foods
- Managing stress through mindfulness and movement
- Staying hydrated and prioritizing sleep

Your gut is more than just a digestive organ—it's the command center of your health. By taking care of it, you're not just improving digestion; you're strengthening your immune system, balancing hormones, and setting the foundation for lifelong well-being.

Signs Your Gut is in Trouble

When Your Gut is Unhappy, It Lets You Know

Your gut is not the silent type. When it's unhappy, it doesn't sit quietly and suffer—it sends distress signals in the form of bloating, skin issues, brain fog, and more. Most people don't connect these symptoms to gut health, but your digestive system plays a huge role in how you feel, think, and even look.

If you've been feeling "off" lately but can't figure out why, your gut might be trying to get your attention. Here are some telltale signs that your gut needs some serious TLC.

1. Digestive Issues: The Most Obvious Red Flag

If your gut isn't happy, your digestion will be the first to suffer. Issues like bloating, gas, constipation, or diarrhea are all signs that something is out of balance.

What's Happening?

- An imbalance in gut bacteria can cause excessive gas and bloating.
- Poor gut health can slow digestion, leading to constipation or speed things up, causing diarrhea.

- Acid reflux and heartburn can also be linked to an unhealthy gut.

If your stomach feels like a balloon after every meal, don't just blame it on bad luck—your gut is struggling.

2. Food Sensitivities: When Your Gut Turns Against You

Do certain foods make you feel sick, bloated, or uncomfortable? You may have food sensitivities—a classic sign of a gut imbalance.

What's Happening?

- A damaged gut lining can make it harder to digest certain foods, leading to bloating, nausea, or cramps.
- An imbalanced microbiome can cause your immune system to overreact to harmless foods.
- Common culprits include dairy, gluten, sugar, and processed foods.

If you feel off after eating certain meals, your gut may be struggling to break down those foods properly.

3. Frequent Illnesses: A Weak Immune System

Did you know that 70% of your immune system is in your gut? If you're constantly sick, your gut health might be to blame.

What's Happening?

- A strong gut microbiome helps train your immune cells to fight infections.
- When your gut is unbalanced, your immune system becomes weaker, making you more prone to colds, flu, and infections.
- Chronic gut inflammation can even contribute to autoimmune diseases.

If you catch every cold that goes around, it's time to show your gut some love.

4. Skin Problems: Your Gut's Struggles Show on Your Face

Acne, eczema, rashes, and even premature aging can be linked to poor gut health.

What's Happening?

- A leaky gut (when your gut lining is damaged) allows toxins into your bloodstream, causing inflammation that shows up on your skin.
- An imbalance of gut bacteria can trigger conditions like acne and eczema.
- Poor digestion means your body isn't absorbing essential nutrients needed for healthy skin.

If expensive skincare products aren't fixing your breakouts, maybe it's time to fix your gut instead.

5. Brain Fog & Mood Swings: When Your Gut Messes with Your Mind

Your gut and brain are tightly connected. If your gut is out of balance, your mood and mental clarity can suffer too.

What's Happening?

- The gut produces 90% of the body's serotonin (the happiness hormone).
- An unhealthy gut can lead to anxiety, mood swings, depression, and brain fog.
- If you often feel sluggish, forgetful, or overwhelmed for no reason, your gut could be affecting your mental health.

How to Keep Your Gut Happy

Now that we understand how important the gut is, let's talk about ways to keep it happy and thriving. A well-balanced gut doesn't just help with digestion — it improves immunity, boosts mood, and even supports glowing skin. So, how do you take care of this microbial wonderland inside you? Follow these gut-friendly habits, and your digestive system will thank you!

1. Eat More Fiber (Your Gut Bugs Will Thank You!)

Fiber is like an all-you-can-eat buffet for your good gut bacteria. They ferment fiber, turning it into beneficial compounds like short-chain fatty acids, which reduce inflammation and improve digestion. The more fiber you eat, the happier your gut bacteria will be!

Best Fiber Sources:

- Fruits & Vegetables: Apples, bananas, berries, spinach, broccoli
- Whole Grains: Oats, brown rice, quinoa
- Legumes: Lentils, chickpeas, beans
- Nuts & Seeds: Chia seeds, flaxseeds, almonds

Pro Tip: Aim for at least 25-30 grams of fiber daily. Your gut will reward you with smooth digestion and less bloating!

Understanding Food Intolerances: Raw Vegetables and Pulses

Many people struggle with digesting raw vegetables or pulses, and this often traces back to an imbalance in the gut microbiome or a deficiency in key digestive enzymes. Raw vegetables and legumes are rich in fiber and complex carbohydrates — components that demand a robust and diverse microbiome for proper digestion. When the gut lacks the necessary bacterial strains or enzymatic activity, these foods can ferment in the digestive tract, leading to symptoms like bloating, gas, cramping, or overall digestive discomfort.

This doesn't mean these foods are inherently bad — on the contrary, they are packed with nutrients, antioxidants, and prebiotic fibers that can support long-term gut health. The issue lies in the gut's current state and its ability to handle these complex plant-based compounds. A weakened or imbalanced microbiome may be the result of a highly processed diet, overuse of antibiotics, chronic stress, or even inadequate hydration — all of which compromise the digestive environment.

The good news? With a mindful approach, it's entirely possible to reintroduce raw vegetables and pulses into the diet and gradually improve gut resilience. Techniques like soaking, sprouting, slow cooking, or fermenting these foods can make them easier to digest initially. Pairing them with digestive aids like ginger, fennel, or cumin can also help stimulate enzyme production and soothe the gut lining.

Additionally, focusing on slowly increasing fiber intake — rather than overwhelming the system all at once — gives the gut time to adapt and encourages the growth of beneficial bacteria. Supplementing with probiotics or incorporating fermented foods such as yogurt, kefir, kimchi, or sauerkraut can further support this microbial diversity.

Ultimately, improving gut health is about consistency, patience, and tuning into your body's signals. With time, many people find they can tolerate — and even thrive on — foods they once struggled with, all thanks to a nourished, better-balanced digestive system.

Raw Vegetables

For those who experience discomfort after eating raw vegetables, the issue often stems from an insufficient population of fiber-digesting bacteria. The solution is to introduce them gradually and support the gut microbiome in adapting.

- **Start with Small Portions:** Introducing small amounts of raw vegetables allows the digestive system to adjust without overwhelming it.
- **Incorporate Fermented Foods:** Fermented vegetables like sauerkraut, kimchi, or pickles provide probiotics that help strengthen gut bacteria, making it easier to digest raw fiber.
- **Opt for Light Cooking:** Steaming or lightly sautéing vegetables softens the fiber while retaining most of the nutrients, making digestion easier.

With time, as the gut adapts, raw vegetables can become a more significant part of the diet without causing discomfort.

Pulses and Legumes

Some people struggle with pulses due to the presence of anti-nutrients and complex carbohydrates that are difficult to digest. This often results in bloating, gas, or an upset stomach. To make them more digestible, certain preparation methods can be helpful.

- **Soaking and Sprouting:** Soaking pulses overnight helps break down phytic acid and other anti-nutrients, making them easier to digest. Sprouting further enhances their nutritional value and reduces digestive discomfort.
- **Proper Cooking Methods:** Pressure cooking or slow cooking helps break down hard-to-digest compounds, making pulses gentler on the stomach.
- **Adding Digestive Spices:** Spices like cumin, ginger, and asafoetida (hing) can aid digestion and reduce bloating, making pulses more tolerable.

By gradually incorporating these methods, individuals can train their digestive systems to handle raw vegetables and pulses more efficiently, ultimately improving gut health and nutrient absorption.

2. Probiotics & Prebiotics: The Dynamic Duo

Prebiotics and probiotics play a crucial role in maintaining gut health, digestion, and immunity. While probiotics are live beneficial bacteria that restore gut balance, prebiotics are fiber-rich foods that feed these bacteria, helping them thrive. Probiotics can be found in fermented foods like yogurt, kefir, kimchi, and traditional Indian staples like buttermilk and kanji, while prebiotics are present in foods such as bananas, garlic, onions, oats, and legumes. Together, they improve digestion, enhance nutrient absorption, reduce bloating, and support metabolism. Many people struggle with digesting raw vegetables or pulses due to a lack of gut bacteria needed to process fiber, making prebiotics essential for building a stronger microbiome.

Your gut is home to trillions of bacteria, and not all of them are bad. To keep the good ones thriving, you need probiotics and prebiotics — the ultimate power couple for gut health.

Probiotics - The Reinforcements Probiotics are live bacteria that boost your gut health by adding more beneficial microbes. Think of them as backup troops for your microbiome.

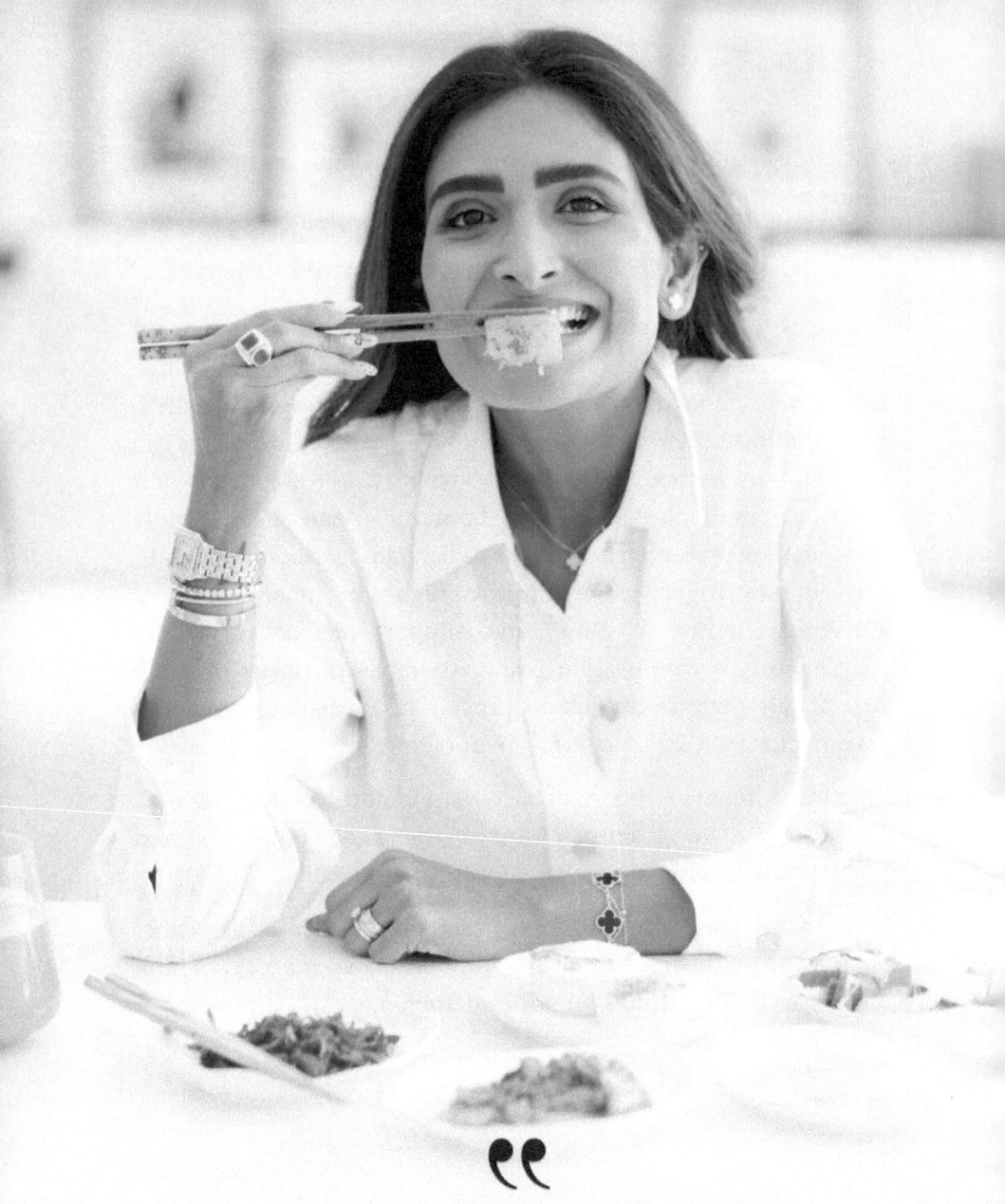

❝ KIMCHI
because sometimes the best things in life are
A LITTLE SOUR, A LITTLE SPICY, AND TOTALLY ALIVE

Best Probiotic Foods:

- Yogurt (with live cultures)
- Kefir
- Sauerkraut & Kimchi
- Miso & Tempeh

Prebiotics – The Food for Your Good Bacteria Prebiotics feed the good bacteria already living in your gut, helping them grow and thrive.

Best Prebiotic Foods:

- Garlic & Onions
- Asparagus
- Bananas
- Oats

Pro Tip: Pair probiotic and prebiotic foods for maximum gut benefits! (Example: Have a bowl of yogurt with bananas and oats.)

3. Cut Back on Gut-Offenders

Just like some foods nourish your gut, others harm it. Eating too many processed or artificial foods can cause gut imbalances, leading to bloating, inflammation, and digestive issues.

- Processed Foods & Sugar – Feeds bad bacteria, causing imbalances.
- Artificial Sweeteners – Can disrupt gut bacteria and cause digestive problems.
- Excessive Alcohol – Damages gut lining and promotes inflammation.
- Unnecessary Antibiotics – Kills both good and bad bacteria, disrupting balance.

Pro Tip: If you must take antibiotics, follow up with probiotics to rebuild your gut bacteria!

Stress vs. Your Gut: The Ultimate Smackdown

If you've ever had butterflies in your stomach before a big event or felt your stomach twist in knots during stress, you've already experienced the gut-brain connection in action. Your gut and brain constantly communicate, and when stress barges in, it throws your digestive system into chaos.

Chronic stress isn't just bad for your mind — it wreaks havoc on your gut microbiome, weakens digestion, and can even cause bloating, stomach cramps, and food intolerances. If your stomach feels off when life gets hectic, stress might be the real culprit.

But don't worry! There are simple, effective ways to calm your nerves and keep your gut happy and balanced.

How Stress Messes with Your Gut

Your gut is often called the "second brain" because it contains millions of neurons that send signals to your brain. When you're stressed, your brain sends panic signals to your gut, which can lead to:

- Slower digestion (causing bloating & constipation)
- Increased stomach acid (leading to heartburn)
- Changes in gut bacteria (triggering inflammation & food sensitivities)

Basically, when you're mentally stressed, your gut feels it physically.

Best Stress-Busting Activities for a Happy Gut

The good news? You can reset your gut-brain connection by managing stress. Here are some science-backed ways to calm your mind and improve digestion:

1. Meditation & Deep Breathing: Even just 5 minutes of meditation or deep breathing can put your body into rest-and-digest mode, improving digestion and reducing gut inflammation.

Try This: Before eating, take three deep breaths to activate your parasympathetic nervous system, which helps your gut work properly.

2. Yoga & Exercise: Physical movement is a powerful stress reliever and also helps your gut function better by improving digestion and reducing bloating.

Best Exercises for Gut Health:

- Yoga Poses like child's pose and twists help with bloating.
- Walking after meals improves digestion.
- Strength training reduces stress hormones.

3. Get Good Sleep (Aim for 7-9 Hours): Poor sleep = increased stress = unhappy gut. Lack of sleep disrupts gut bacteria, making you more prone to inflammation and digestion issues.

Better Sleep Tips:

- No screens one hour before bed (blue light messes with melatonin).
- Keep your bedroom cool and dark.
- Try herbal teas like chamomile for relaxation.

4. Spend Time in Nature: Nature has a magical way of reducing stress and balancing gut bacteria. Fresh air, sunshine, and walking barefoot on grass can lower cortisol (the stress hormone) and improve digestion.

Try This: Take a 10-minute walk outside every day — it does wonders for your gut!

Hydration: Don't Forget the Basics

Water is like oil for your digestive engine — without enough of it, everything slows down, leading to bloating, constipation, and sluggish digestion. Staying hydrated helps your gut absorb nutrients, break down food, and flush out waste efficiently. Think of your gut as a highway — without water, traffic jams (aka constipation) are inevitable!

How Much Water Do You Need?

Aim for at least 8 glasses (2 liters) of water per day, but if you're active or live in a hot climate, you may need more.

Bonus Tip: Start your morning with warm lemon water! It hydrates your body, kickstarts digestion, and supports your liver in detoxifying overnight waste.

Signs You're Not Drinking Enough Water:

- Constipation or hard stools
- Dry skin and lips
- Feeling fatigued or sluggish
- Frequent bloating

Staying hydrated is one of the simplest and most effective ways to keep your gut happy. So, grab that water bottle and sip your way to better digestion!

Treat Your Gut Like a VIP

I spent most of my life thinking that bloating, fatigue, and random breakouts were just *normal*. I had always been told I had a "weak stomach" and that certain foods — like dairy and wheat — would "strengthen" me. So, I kept eating them, even when I felt terrible afterward. I ignored the discomfort, the sluggishness, the constant brain fog, because I didn't know any better.

Doctors prescribed medications, family members suggested home remedies, and I tried every probiotic or "gut-healing" supplement I could find. But nothing really helped. It wasn't until I started researching on my own that I realized the foods I was told to eat— the ones that were supposed to nourish me—were the ones actually hurting me. Dairy, gluten, and processed foods weren't just minor irritants; they were triggering inflammation, messing with my digestion, and weakening my immunity.

The more I learned, the more it all made sense. My gut wasn't just struggling; it was *crying for help*. I had been ignoring the symptoms, brushing them off as stress or genetics, when in reality, my body had been fighting a battle I didn't even know I was waging.

So, I made changes. I started cutting out the foods that triggered my symptoms, added gut-friendly alternatives, and focused on whole, unprocessed meals. It wasn't an overnight fix, but within weeks, I noticed something different—I wasn't bloated all the time. My skin started clearing up. I felt lighter, more energetic. And for the first time in years, I didn't feel *trapped* in my own body.

This journey taught me that gut health isn't just about digestion — it's about everything. The way you feel, the energy you have, your skin, your mood, even your immune system — it all connects back to the gut. And the best part? You have control over it.

If you've been struggling with bloating, fatigue, constant breakouts, or unexplained health issues, don't just accept it as your "normal." Listen to your body. Start paying attention to what makes you feel good and what makes you feel worse.

Because once you start healing your gut, you start healing *everything*. And trust me, the difference is life-changing.

Your gut isn't just a food-processing factory—it's a control center for your entire body. A happy gut means better digestion, stronger immunity, improved mood, and even glowing skin.

By feeding it the right foods, cutting out harmful ones, and managing stress, you'll be rewarded with better health and more energy. So, the next time you sit down for a meal, remember: you're not just feeding yourself—you're feeding trillions of tiny bacteria inside you. Treat them well!

Conclusion

As we reach the final pages of *Nourish Without Nonsense*, I hope this book has provided you with a fresh perspective on health, nutrition, and the importance of understanding your own body. My journey — from childhood struggles with digestion to years of misinformation, trial and error, and eventual clarity — has been deeply personal, yet I know I am not alone. So many people today feel lost in the maze of conflicting dietary advice, food fads, and restrictive meal plans that only lead to frustration rather than true health.

The biggest lesson I have learned — and the message I want to leave you with — is that nourishment should never feel like a burden. Eating well, feeling good, and living a vibrant life should not come with guilt, confusion, or stress. Instead, it should be a joyful, intuitive, and fulfilling process.

We have been conditioned to believe that health requires extreme measures — cutting out entire food groups, subscribing to rigid diet plans, or punishing our bodies with unrealistic fitness routines. But the truth is, the most effective approach to health is often the simplest. It's about:

- Listening to your body and recognizing what truly nourishes it.
- Prioritizing whole, unprocessed foods without obsessing over perfection.
- Finding movement that feels enjoyable rather than forced.
- Learning to eat mindfully and with appreciation rather than restriction.
- Understanding that health is a lifelong journey, not a quick fix.

In today's world, health and nutrition are often overcomplicated by trends and conflicting advice. We've been conditioned to believe that achieving good health requires extreme measures and rigid plans. However, the true path to nourishment lies in simplicity — **back to the roots**. Instead of constantly testing new diets, step back and embrace whole, unprocessed foods, listen to your body, and prioritize mindful eating. Health is not about perfection or quick fixes. It's about creating balance, fostering well-being, and rediscovering the natural, intuitive way to nourish your body — back to the roots, where nourishment was truly without nonsense.

Breaking Free from the Chains of Food Guilt

For too long, food has been associated with guilt, discipline, and deprivation. We've been told that certain foods are 'good' and others are 'bad,' creating an unhealthy relationship with eating. The truth is, food is neither an enemy nor a reward. It is simply fuel — meant to nourish, energize, and satisfy. By redefining our mindset, we can break free from food guilt and embrace a healthier, more intuitive way of eating.

Rather than focusing on what you can't have, shift your focus to what you can add — nutrient-dense foods, mindful eating habits, and a sense of enjoyment in the process. The goal is not to follow a rigid plan but to build a lifestyle that supports your health while allowing for flexibility and joy.

One of the most common mistakes people make when trying to improve their health is expecting drastic results overnight. But true transformation comes from small, sustainable changes over time. Instead of overhauling your diet in one go, start with manageable shifts:

- Swap out processed snacks for whole food alternatives.
- Hydrate more consistently.
- Incorporate gut-friendly foods.
- Move your body in a way that feels natural to you.

- Practice mindful eating and portion awareness.

These small actions, when repeated consistently, create lasting results. There's no need for an all-or-nothing approach — progress is built on daily choices, not fleeting moments of perfection.

Reclaiming Your Health — On Your Own Terms

Throughout this book, I have shared insights into gut health, the right portions of nutrients, detox and fasting, and the power of circadian rhythm. But ultimately, none of it matters if it doesn't resonate with you. The real power lies in understanding what works best for your body and making choices that support your personal health goals.

You are the expert on your own body. You don't need to follow trends, succumb to diet culture, or adopt extreme measures just because they work for someone else. Your health journey is yours — and that means it should be enjoyable, sustainable, and aligned with your lifestyle.

A common struggle that many people face is the fear of making the 'wrong' choice when it comes to food. We are bombarded with conflicting advice — one day, a certain food is deemed a superfood, and the next, it's labeled harmful. This overwhelming flood of information creates anxiety around eating. But let me remind you: health is not about perfection. It's about balance.

Instead of chasing an unattainable ideal, focus on the bigger picture. Ask yourself:

- Do I feel energized after eating?
- Am I nourishing my body with a variety of nutrients?
- Do I enjoy my meals without guilt or stress?

When you start measuring success based on how you feel rather than how closely you adhere to rigid rules, you will find a newfound sense of freedom in your health journey.

The Power of Mindful Eating

One of the simplest yet most powerful habits you can develop is mindful eating. In today's fast-paced world, we often eat on autopilot—scrolling through our phones, rushing through meals, or eating out of boredom rather than hunger. By slowing down and paying attention to our food, we can develop a healthier relationship with eating.

Mindful eating involves:

- Eating without distractions.
- Tuning into hunger and fullness cues.
- Savoring each bite and appreciating the flavors.
- Recognizing emotional eating patterns and addressing them with self-compassion.

When we practice mindfulness with food, we become more attuned to what our bodies need. We naturally begin to eat in a way that supports our well-being rather than relying on external rules to dictate our choices.

Moving Forward with Confidence

As you close this book, I want you to move forward with confidence. You now have the knowledge and tools to nourish yourself without nonsense—without confusion, unnecessary stress, or external pressure. You have everything you need to thrive, and the power to make mindful, informed choices is in your hands.

Let this be the beginning of a new chapter, one where you embrace health as a celebration rather than a struggle. Trust yourself, be patient with your journey, and remember: health is not about perfection—it's about feeling your best, every day, in a way that works for you.

This book is not just about changing what you eat—it's about changing your perspective on food, health, and self-care. It's about rejecting diet culture, freeing yourself from unnecessary stress, and stepping into a life where wellness feels natural and effortless.

Your Next Steps

As you embark on this journey, here are some practical steps to keep in mind:

1. **Start where you are.** You don't need to have everything figured out. Just take one step at a time.
2. **Keep it simple.** Don't overcomplicate things. Focus on whole, nourishing foods and find an approach that feels natural to you.
3. **Keep experimenting.** Health is not one-size-fits-all. Stay open to learning what works best for you.
4. **Be kind to yourself.** There will be days when you don't eat as well as you'd like, and that's okay. Progress is about consistency, not perfection.
5. **Celebrate small wins.** Every healthy choice you make is a step toward a better you.
6. **Stay curious.** Continue learning, trying new foods, and evolving your approach to wellness.

Thank you for allowing me to be part of your journey. Writing this book has been an incredible experience, and my greatest hope is that it serves as a source of encouragement, inspiration, and practical guidance for you.

Remember, health is not a destination—it's a journey. And that journey should be filled with nourishment, joy, and balance.

Here's to a life of nourishment, balance, and true wellness—without the nonsense.

Acknowledgements

Writing Nourish Without Nonsense has been a journey of both reflection and resilience, and I'm deeply grateful for everyone who walked alongside me as this book came to life.

To my readers — thank you for trusting me with your time, curiosity, and most importantly, your health. You are the reason this book exists. My hope is that these pages remind you that nourishment can be simple, powerful, and rooted in self-respect.

To my family, whose unconditional love and belief in me have been the foundation of everything I do — thank you for always reminding me of my purpose. Your support, late-night pep talks, and taste-testing skills were invaluable.

To my clients and community — your stories, struggles, and wins have inspired every chapter. You taught me that healing isn't linear and that progress, no matter how small, is worth celebrating.

To my incredible team and editor - your unwavering commitment, sharp insight, and behind the scene brilliance made this book not only possible but better. I'm endlessly thankful for your patience, precision and passion throughout the process.

To my mentors and fellow health professionals — thank you for pushing me to stay grounded in both science and compassion. Your guidance has shaped my philosophy and my voice.

And finally, to anyone who's ever felt overwhelmed by conflicting food rules or disconnected from their body — this book was written for you. May it be your permission slip to unlearn the noise and return to what truly nourishes you.

With all my gratitude,
Saanchi

Let's Stay Connected

Your journey doesn't end with the last page. Join our growing community for gut-friendly recipes, real talk about wellness, and daily doses of encouragement. I'd love to hear how Nourish Without Nonsense has impacted your life — share your thoughts, tag me, or just drop a hello!

- Instagram: @thesaanchishetty / @saanchishetty9
- Facebook/X/Youtube: @thesaanchishetty
- Website: www.thesaanchishetty.com

Let's keep nourishing — without the nonsense. 🤍

www.ingramcontent.com/pod-product-compliance
Lightning Source LLC
LaVergne TN
LVHW041909070526
838199LV00051BA/2558